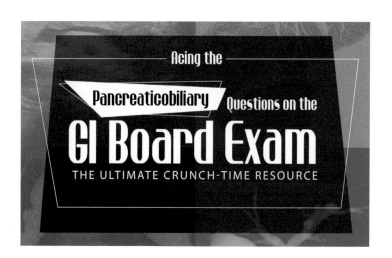

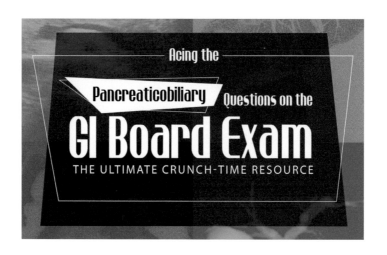

Acing the **Pancreaticobiliary** Questions on the **GI Board Exam**
THE ULTIMATE CRUNCH-TIME RESOURCE

Authors

Brennan M. R. Spiegel, MD, MSHS, FACG, AGAF
Editor-in-Chief, *American Journal of Gastroenterology*
Professor of Medicine and Public Health
Director of Health Services Research
Cedars-Sinai Medical Center
Los Angeles, California

Hetal A. Karsan, MD, FACG, FASGE, FAASLD, FACP
Editor of the Red Section and Associate Editor
American Journal of Gastroenterology
Adjunct Professor of Medicine
Division of Digestive Diseases and Emory Transplant Center
Emory University School of Medicine
Atlanta Gastroenterology Associates
Atlanta, Georgia

Contributing Editor

Tilak Shah, MD, MHS
Director of Interventional Endoscopy
Hunter Holmes McGuire VA Medical Center
Assistant Professor of Medicine
Virginia Commonwealth University
Richmond, Virginia

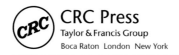
CRC Press
Taylor & Francis Group
Boca Raton   London   New York

CRC Press is an imprint of the
Taylor & Francis Group, an **informa** business

First published in 2018 by SLACK Incorporated

Published 2024 by CRC Press
2385 NW Executive Center Drive, Suite 320, Boca Raton FL 33431

and by CRC Press
4 Park Square, Milton Park, Abingdon, Oxon, OX14 4RN

CRC Press is an imprint of Taylor & Francis Group, LLC

Library of Congress Cataloging-in-Publication Data

Names: Spiegel, Brennan M. R., 1972- author. | Karsan, Hetal A., 1971-
    author. | Shah, Tilak, author.
Title: Acing the pancreaticobiliary questions on the GI Board Exam : the
    ultimate crunch-time resource / authors, Brennan MR Spiegel, Hetal A
    Karsan ; contributing author, Tilak Shah.
Description: Thorofare, NJ : SLACK Incorporated, [2018] | Includes
    bibliographical references and index.
Identifiers: LCCN 2017040574| ISBN 9781630911188 (pbk. : alk. paper) |

Subjects: | MESH: Pancreatic Diseases | Biliary Tract Diseases | Examination
    Questions
Classification: LCC RC858.P35 | NLM WI 18.2 | DDC 616.3/70076--dc23 LC record available at
https://lccn.loc.gov/2017040574

ISBN: 9781630911188 (hbk)
ISBN: 9781003522478 (ebk)

DOI: 10.1201/9781003522478

DEDICATION

To Shelly Lu for directing a world class Gastroenterology & Hepatology Division at Cedars-Sinai that enables its faculty to advance science and education in all facets of our field. To Shlomo Melmed and Scott Weingarten for the privilege of working at Cedars-Sinai under their expert leadership and support. A book like this is only possible with a nurturing, supportive, and academically focused environment.

And as always, to my loving wife and children who continue to put up with me working too much on books like this one.

—Brennan M. R. Spiegel, MD, MSHS, FACG, AGAF

To my colleagues at Atlanta Gastroenterology Associates, Emory University and former students, residents, fellows, and friends whose ongoing feedback continues to make me feel assured that I am providing an effective and tangible educational service amid the vast, limitless universe of knowledge to be acquired.

And most importantly, to my precious wife, Lina, and beloved children, Rajan and Sonia, for all of their steadfast support and inspiration. These books would not have been possible without them.

Iamque opus exegi. Om Shanti Shanti Shanti.

—Hetal A. Karsan, MD, FACG, FASGE, FAASLD, FACP

CONTENTS

ACKNOWLEDGMENTS

The authors wish to thank the following physicians who provided images for this book:

- Vaidehi Avadhani, MD, Emory University
- Joel Camilo, MD, Atlanta Gastroenterology Associates
- Bruce T. Kalmin, MD, Atlanta Gastroenterology Associates
- Nandhakumar Kanagarajan, MD, Atlanta Gastroenterology Associates
- Divyanshoo R. Kohli, MD, Mayo Clinic Arizona
- Jamie B. MacKelfresh, MD, Emory University
- Courtney Moreno, MD, Emory University
- Jung Suh, MD, MPH, Atlanta Gastroenterology Associates
- Robert A. Swerlick, MD, Emory University

ABOUT THE AUTHORS

Brennan M. R. Spiegel, MD, MSHS, FACG, AGAF is Professor of Medicine, Director of Health Services Research, and Director of the Master's Degree Program in Health Delivery Science at Cedars-Sinai Medical Center. He is the Editor-in-Chief of the *American Journal of Gastroenterology*.

Dr. Spiegel attended Tufts University where he majored in philosophy and community health, and received his MD with Alpha Omega Alpha honors from New York Medical College. He received training in internal medicine at Cedars-Sinai Medical Center in Los Angeles, completed a fellowship in gastroenterology at UCLA, where he developed the material for the *Acing* books while studying for Boards, and completed advanced studies in health services research at the UCLA School of Public Health, where he received a master's degree in health services. He received a Research Career Development Award through the Veteran Administration (VA) during which time he was trained in health services methodology.

Dr. Spiegel's research interests have focused on functional GI disorders, IBDs, acid-peptic disorders, chronic liver disease, GI hemorrhage, and colon cancer screening. He also studies the role of digital health technologies in clinical practice, including patient-provider portals, social media analytics, wearable biosensors, and therapeutic virtual reality. His research has been funded by the National Institutes of Health, VA, Robert Wood Johnson Foundation, Hearst Foundation, Patient Centered Outcomes Research Institute (PCORI), California Initiative for the Advancement of Precision Medicine, The Marc and Sheri Rapaport Fund for Digital Health Sciences & Precision Health, and the American College of Gastroenterology, among other sources.

Hetal A. Karsan, MD, FACG, FASGE, FAASLD, FACP is an Adjunct Professor of Medicine in the Division of Diseases at Emory University School of Medicine. He practices as a clinical gastroenterologist, hepatologist, and partner at Atlanta Gastroenterology Associates and also maintains a clinical practice at Emory University. He is the Editor of the Red Section and Associate Editor of the *American Journal of Gastroenterology*.

Dr. Karsan attended Indiana University, where he earned his bachelor of science in biology and won awards from the Howard Hughes Medical Institute for undergraduate biomedical research. He obtained his doctor of medicine from the Indiana University School of Medicine. Thereafter, he received training in internal medicine at Boston University, where he completed his medical internship and residency and also served as acting Chief Medical Resident. He went on to complete his fellowship at UCLA Medical Center, where he trained in gastroenterology, advanced interventional endoscopy, and transplant hepatology. While at UCLA, he also pursued advanced clinical research training through the UCLA School of Public Health. He is Board-certified in internal medicine, gastroenterology, and transplant hepatology.

Dr. Karsan is active in a number of professional organizations and editorial boards. He is Board-certified in internal medicine, gastroenterology, and transplant hepatology and actively participates in clinical outcomes research. In his leisure time, he enjoys sports, traveling, baking, and spending time with his family.

ABOUT THE CONTRIBUTING EDITOR

Tilak Shah, MD, MHS is the Director of Interventional Endoscopy at the Hunter Holmes McGuire VA Medical Center in Richmond, Virginia, and Assistant Professor of Medicine in the Division of Gastroenterology at Virginia Commonwealth University. He completed his residency and fellowship training at Duke University Medical Center, where he also pursued a master's degree in clinical research. Subsequently, he attained specialized training in interventional endoscopy at Emory University and has published several clinical studies related to pancreaticobiliary disorders.

PREFACE

Before we get started, take a look at this map of the United States:

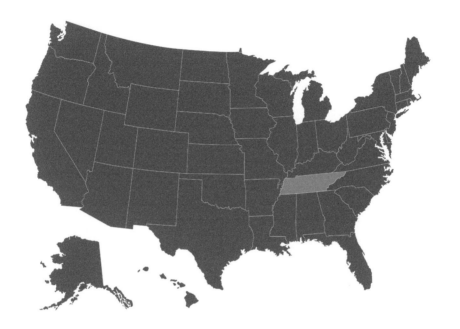

You'll notice that the state of Tennessee is highlighted right in the middle of the map. What makes Tennessee special? Probably a lot of things. But here's an interesting fact about Tennessee: it's tied with Missouri for bordering more states than any other state in the Union. In fact, Tennessee touches 8 other states along its expansive border. Tennessee leads the state neighbor competition for 2 reasons: it's landlocked, so all its borders share territory with neighboring states; and it's long and thin, spanning great distance and boasting a large surface area for such a diminutive landmass (ranked #36) and population (ranked #17). Tennessee may be small, but it packs a punch and topographically anchors a huge part of the nation. If foreign invaders wanted to quickly occupy the United States, they'd be wise to start from Tennessee and work their way out. Before long, marauding troops would be in everyone's backyards.

So, what's this got anything to do with a book about the pancreas? Sort of everything. You see, Tennessee is a lot like the pancreas. For starters, both are shaped similarly, each with a head, a tail, and protracted length in between. They're also both landlocked. The pancreas lies deep within the retroperitoneum, shrouded along all its borders with viscera, vessels, and connective tissue. For an organ that isn't very big, the pancreas gets all up in everybody's business: it borders the stomach, biliary tree, spleen, duodenum, aorta, portal vein, splenic vein, and left kidney (just so happens to be 8 major structures). Take a look:

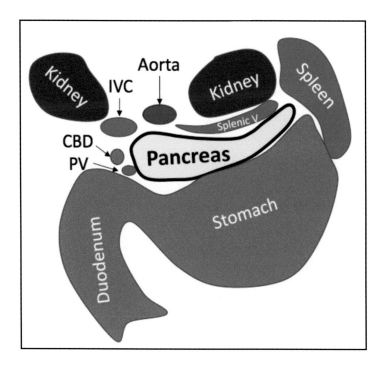

If a bomb goes off in the pancreas, then the whole body learns about it real fast. The pancreas can wreak havoc, not only upon its immediate neighbors, but also through a cascade of damage propagating throughout the body. Like Tennessee, the pancreas has a disproportionately high surface area, touches all sorts of vital neighbors, invests itself in critical local functions with broad effects, and when "invaded" or otherwise perturbed, can send toxic emissaries out quickly and efficiently through land (ie local viscera), sea (ie blood vessels), and air (ie respiratory and alimentary tracts). So, we've got to take the pancreas very seriously and protect it at all costs.

This book is all about the pancreas. It's also about those tubes running alongside and through the pancreas—ie the biliary tree. To extend this crazy analogy, we'll call the biliary tree the "Mississippi River" of the pancreas, running along its Western border. In this book, the fourth in the *Acing the GI Board Exam* series of review manuals, we'll explore how the pancreas can be invaded, perturbed, or otherwise become toxic. We'll also review how its great tributaries—the biliary tree and pancreatic duct—can become blocked, dammed up, overflowed, or otherwise rerouted, naturally or by purposeful intervention; and we'll do it while having fun through our patented "Acing the Boards" style of unhinged pedagogy (as this inane introduction demonstrates).

The first book in the *Acing* series, entitled *Acing the GI Board Exam: The Ultimate Crunch-Time Resource*, sampled from the breadth and depth of topics that could be encountered on the American Board of Internal Medicine (ABIM) GI Examination. The second book, entitled *Acing the Hepatology Questions on the GI Board Exam*, focused exclusively on liver diseases, and was the first of a series of topic-focused reviews designed to complement the original *Acing* book. The third book covered inflammatory bowel disease (IBD) in depth. We now introduce our latest edition to the *Acing* series with this review of pancreaticobiliary (ie "panc-bil") topics. Similar to hepatology and IBD, it is hard to keep up with the burgeoning panc-bil literature. Until now, there has been no single, slim, but high-yield volume that summarizes the panc-bil topics you really need to know for the Boards. We think this book nailed it. We collected every pearl of wisdom, high-yield factlet, panc-bil "Board buzzword," and classic imaging study we could muster, all while keeping the book a manageable size.

The first 3 *Acing* books included a wide variety of panc-bil questions. Here, we provide new questions to round out the panc-bil content for everyday practice as well as preparing for the Board examination. We minimized content overlap among the books to ensure this volume is unique from its predecessors. Between the 4 books in the expanded *Acing* series, we now cover every major topic in panc-bil, with a focus on the "tough stuff" vignettes you may not know the answer to (yet).

We've made every effort to write a modern, up-to-date, panc-bil textbook. But we're also cognizant that the Board exam focuses on "prime time" knowledge—not recent insights or evolving hypotheses. In preparing this book, we sought to strike a balance between interesting stuff you should know about in clinical practice, and high-yield stuff that might actually appear on a Board exam. These are not the same.

Although we have many years of clinical experience, including Hetal Karsan's interventional endoscopy training at UCLA, we wanted even more experience in order to produce a first-rate book. Thus, in addition to stalwarts Brennan Spiegel and Hetal Karsan, who scribed earlier volumes in the *Acing* series, here we add Tilak Shah as a key contributor. Dr. Shah completed residency and fellowship training at Duke University, interventional endoscopy training at Emory, and has published several panc-bil manuscripts. He is currently the Director of interventional endoscopy at the Hunter Holmes McGuire VA Medical Center and an assistant professor at Virginia Commonwealth University.

The remainder of the Preface, below, explains how the *Acing* approach works, and how we try to get you where you need to be without going too far. We maintained the same Preface that appears in the other *Acing* books, since the content is just as relevant to panc-bil as it is to general GI and hepatology. In the following chapter, entitled Panc-Bil on the GI Board Exam, we discuss issues specific to panc-bil, and describe how the current book aims to focus on panc-bil knowledge of relevance to the general gastroenterologist.

At this point in your career you know a lot. It's been a hard-earned battle, but after years of reading books, sitting through lectures, and working with patients, you now have a pretty good sense of what's important and what's, well, less important. You're also busy, and your time is limited. So now that you want to quickly review the important topics in gastroenterology or have to study for Boards or prepare for a clerkship, your goal is to learn the stuff you don't know, not review the stuff you already do know.

Yet, for some reason, we all continue to practice an inefficient approach to studying for Board exams. This usually consists of comprehensively reviewing the entirety of a topic area without thinking about (a) whether we're adding incremental information to our pre-existing storehouse of knowledge, and (b) whether we're learning things that may actually come up on the examination. Presumably you've already done the painstaking work of learning the basics of your trade. Now you've got to get to business and ace a test. Those are 2 very different activities.

Yet, the inefficient approach to Board review is perennially fostered by traditional Board review textbooks, in which content areas are laid out in chapter-by-chapter (and verse) detail, fully laden with facts both high and low yield—both relevant and irrelevant to actual examinations. There's a time and place for the chapter and verse approach to learning your trade, but Board review crunch-time probably isn't it.

But Board review books usually go a step further. They often present information that is not important in preparation for the Boards (and very unlikely to appear on the Boards), but that is merely of personal interest to the chapter authors. That is, many Board review books suffer from the affliction of academia running roughshod over practical information. This stuff is usually prefaced by the standard forerunners, like "Recent data indicate that… " or "Our group recently discovered that… " or "Although there is still a lack of consensus that… " and so forth. This kind of information is interesting and important for so many reasons, but is not for Board review. When you're in crunch-time, you shouldn't have to read about pet theories, areas of utter controversy (and thus ineligible for Board exams), or brand new or incompletely tested data that is too immature for Board exams. You need to know about time-tested pearls that are more likely to appear —not cutting-edge hypotheses, novel speculations, new epidemiological oddities, or anything else not yet ready for prime time. Board exams are about prime time.

The *Acing* books are different. Even if you aren't taking a Board exam, we have created concise power review manuals for you. They aim for the sweet spot between what you already know, and what you don't already know (or forgot)—which may or may not appear on the Boards. They try to avoid the lower extreme of stuff you've known since birth, and the upper extreme of academic ruminations that are great for journal club or staying on the cutting edge, but probably sit on the cutting room floor in Board exam editorial offices. You may find that you do know some of the stuff in this book, and if so, that's great. That means you're almost ready for the exam. But you'll also find that you don't know (or have forgotten) much of this book. And that's the point—you should be reading stuff you don't know, not reviewing content you already know well. We've filled this book with stuff you probably don't know. Heck, even we need to read this book from time-to-time to remember this stuff.

The information in this book is culled from years of clinical practice experience and teaching Board review to our gastroenterology fellows and students. We've come to realize that our fellows and colleagues in community practice, who are amongst the best of the best, know a lot about their specialty, but are not necessarily ready for Boards. That's because we purposefully do not teach for Boards during everyday training—we instead teach the skills and knowledge that support rational and evidence-based decision-making in clinical practice. Unfortunately, Board exams don't always tap directly into those skill sets. Great clinicians can do poorly on Board exams. And great test-takers can be suboptimal clinicians. We all recognize that it's primarily important to be a great clinician, and secondarily important to be a great test-taker.

But with that caveat, it's still important to ace the Boards. And acing the Boards means that you ace, not only the stuff you know, but also the "tough stuff" you may not yet know. Although it's not ethical or legal to copy Board exam material, there are basic content areas that are likely to show up on these exams. We've tried to predict what these content areas will be based on our clinical experiences and our own longstanding experience teaching Board review classes, including our annual in-person live *Acing the GI Board Exam* review course.

This book consists of a series of high yield vignettes on favorite topics, generally on the more difficult side, and full of pearls that may come in handy come Board time or when you are seeing patients in a clinical setting. All of these are original—none are from an actual Board exam, naturally. But all have been reviewed, through an ongoing process of content development including our annual *Acing the GI Board Exam* symposium. It goes without saying that we have no idea what will be on your Board exam—and even if we did, we're sure as heck not going to give you the answers in a book! Instead, we can make the more general statement that the stuff in this book is probably in the ballpark of things you should know to help you on the exam. More importantly, this will help serve as a concise review for you.

Here are some highlights of this book:

- **Focus on clinical vignettes.** We see actual patients in clinical practice, and, to the Board's credit, most Board questions are clinical vignettes, which makes sense. This book presents questions in the form of clinical vignettes, not sterile, fact-laden blocks of text.

- **Relatively short.** Most Board review books are better suited for arm-curls than for rapidly and effectively teaching their content. Said another way, they're not "bathroom reading." Instead, most Board review books are read at a desk with a highlighter in hand. Unlike traditional didactic volumes, this book is big-time bathroom reading. You know, you sit down, open it up, and take in high-yield "tough stuff" in a hopefully entertaining format in short order. Depending on your Bristol Stool Type, you might get through 1 vignette (ie if you're Bristol 7), or maybe 5 to 10 vignettes (ie Bristol 1). This is not a definitive text for comprehensive Board review, but a one-stop shop for high-impact stuff presented in a novel and interactive way. This book can be used in concert with longer volumes if you're looking for more extensive topic coverage. That said, with the arrival of this latest book, the combination of all 4 *Acing* books (original, hepatology, IBD, panc-bil) now provides a truly comprehensive review of gastroenterology and hepatology. For even more, you can go to our online *Acing* question bank (www.acingboardexams.com) or come to our annual live course.

- **Focus on stuff you don't know.** The goal of this book is for you to learn new stuff on every page, not to rehash stuff you already know. This book is relatively short—but it's dense with material you may not know yet. That's the point—learn stuff you don't know yet, don't keep reading and rereading stuff you've known forever.

- **Emphasis on pearl after pearl after pearl.** Everyone loves clinical pearls. And so do the Boards. After every vignette in this book there's a pearl explicitly stated at the bottom. We call these "Here's the Point!" Know them well. In fact, you will have gained so many pearls that you will be able to make a necklace.

- **Random order of vignettes.** The Boards present questions in random order, not in nice, neat chapters. This book is meant to emulate the Board experience by providing vignettes in random order. It's a way to introduce cognitive dissonance into your learning by constantly switching directions. After all, patients appear in random order, so why not Board review material? If there's a specific topic you want to review, then you can check out the index and find the relevant pages. But again, keep in mind that this is not meant to be a treatise on any single topic, but instead a rapid-fire review of high-yield content.

- **Few multiple-choice questions.** Multiple-choice questions are usually boring. They often test process of elimination more than knowledge and aptitude. When we teach Board review, we typically present a vignette, and then ask: "So what next?" or "What treatment will you give?" It's more entertaining and realistic. When patients come into an office, they don't have a multiple-choice grid floating over their head in a hologram. So we find open-ended questions to be more engaging and interesting, even if the Boards emphasize a multiple-choice format. Believe us, if you can get these questions right without multiple-choice, then you'll most definitely get them right with multiple-choice. There are other sources for straight-up multiple-choice question banks, such as our *Acing* online website: www.acingboardexams.com.

- **Emphasis on "Clinical Thresholds."** We made up this idea of a "Clinical Threshold" after years of clinical practice and teaching Board review. The idea is that there are many Board questions that require the test-taker to memorize some numerical threshold value. Like "So long as an ampullary adenoma is < 2 to 3 cm in size, and assuming there are no lymph nodes on imaging or extension of the tumor into the ductal systems on EUS, endoscopic ampullectomy remains a treatment option." And so forth. These are emphasized throughout the vignettes.

- **Comprehensive yet parsimonious explanations.** Some books provide multiple-choice questions and only give the letter answer without an explanation. Other books only provide a tiny explanation. Others provide a full explanation, but with information that is not relevant. We've even found books that provide a full explanation that is downright wrong! This book tries to provide a comprehensive (and factually correct) answer to a non–multiple-choice question while keeping it succinct and emphasizing the key clinical pearls. In other words, it attempts to give enough information to understand how to answer the question correctly without overwhelming the reader with additional details or misleading information. Board review is not about ruminating forever about personal areas of interest—it's about cutting to the chase and keeping information on target.

- **Avoidance of mind-numbing prose.** Too many review books are boring as heck. They take away our will to live. We wrote this book as inoculation against the painful affliction of Board preparation. In fact, during production of our first 3 *Acing* books, a professional editor heavily altered our text by removing contractions and other writing informalities—we switched it all back again! This isn't *The Canterbury Tales*! This is Board review time, baby! It's already painful enough to open a book and read. Let's make it halfway interesting, light, and hopefully a little humorous (we do our best… bear with us). We've tried to include interesting vignettes, provide answers that draw from "real-life" clinical experience, and avoid unnecessary jargon or excessive academic descriptions.

- **Emphasis on images.** Clinical medicine is a visual art. And panc-bil is often a visual subspecialty. The Boards acknowledge this by including lots of questions with images. Many of the vignettes in this book are accompanied by a carefully selected image designed to bring the content to life and aid in understanding the key points of the case.

This book was greatly enhanced by the feedback and input from current and former GI fellows at Cedars-Sinai Medical Center and colleagues at Atlanta Gastroenterology Associates and Emory University. We remain especially grateful to Benjamin Weinberg, who helped develop the title of the original *Acing the GI Board Exam* book, of which this is the fourth in the series. We'd also like to again thank the physicians mentioned earlier in the acknowledgments, who provided images to help reinforce the clinical content of this book. These images greatly enhance the visual appeal and pedagogy of the text, and for that we are greatly appreciate these experts' time and effort in improving the book.

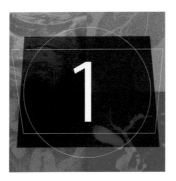

PANC-BIL ON THE
GI BOARD EXAM

As mentioned in the Preface, we have no idea what will show up on your Board exam. Moreover, we don't know about specific vignettes that have appeared on past exams. We only know about general content areas that seem to be popular for Board review, and others that seem to be relatively de-emphasized. Of course, this might all change next year—past isn't always prologue. But with that caveat, here are some observations about general panc-bil topics that we emphasize in Board review:

- **Acute pancreatitis and its complications.** You just know that acute pancreatitis is going to be emphasized on any GI examination. You'll practically have pancreatitis yourself by the time you finish. So, spare yourself a "panc ache" during the test and learn all about acute pancreatitis and its complications. A ripe area to study is the algorithm for managing pancreatic necrosis, as outlined in the American College of Gastroenterology (ACG) pancreatitis guidelines. Know how to manage acute peripancreatic fluid collections and walled off pancreatic necrosis, also called WOPN. See our "WhOPpiN' Pain" vignette in the book for a full run down on this algorithm and its nuances. Examples of nuance: How does the presence of a pancreatic pseudoaneurysm affect how to manage WOPN? How does clinical stability affect your management plan? And so forth. Of course, there are other complications to know about, including pancreatic pseudocysts, pancreaticopleural fistulae, and so forth. Know, for example, that the previous dictum to drain a pseudocyst > 6 cm or persisting > 6 weeks after pancreatitis is old school—you don't drain those, unless the patient is symptomatic. Know that the initial treatment of pancreaticopleural fistula is pancreatic stent placement.

Spiegel BMR, Karsan HA.
Acing the Pancreaticobiliary Questions on the GI Board Exam:
The Ultimate Crunch-Time Resource (pp 1-4).
© 2018 Taylor & Francis Group.

- **Cholangiograms.** Oh yeah, learn those cholangiograms because it'll serve you well. There are a bunch of classics. You should also brush up on the pancreatograms while you are at it. Be ready to identify pancreas divisum, annular pancreas ("double bubble sign"), all the biliary cysts (particularly types I to III), recurrent pyogenic cholangitis (look for biliary stones with an empty gallbladder), pancreatic head cancer ("double duct sign"), and anomalous panc-bil junction, or APBJ. Know how to manage these, too. We've included examples of all the classics throughout the book.

- **Pancreas cysts and neoplasms.** This is another eminently testable area full of Board review "buzzwords." What if we were to say a cyst looks like a "honeycomb?" Or a "cluster of grapes?" Which pancreas cyst has a central scar? Which has a fish mouth ampulla (you know that one, right?). Which cyst has branched finger-like projections on cytology? Which are more common in men? In women? In young people? And so forth. We've summarized all the cysts in our "Name that Cyst!" series of vignettes, and display the key facts in a table you should just memorize like crazy.

- **Inherited conditions that affect the pancreas.** There are a bunch of highly testable inherited conditions that can affect the pancreas. We highlight these conditions elsewhere in the *Acing* series, but also reinforce them throughout this book and introduce new ones as well. For example, you should know what FAMMM is and its associated genetic mutation, CDKN2A. Be familiar with inherited causes of pancreatitis, including hereditary pancreatitis (PRSS-1 mutation), autosomal recessive hereditary pancreatitis (SPINK1), and Peutz-Jeghers syndrome (STK11). There are also childhood conditions that can affect the pancreas, including cystic fibrosis (CFTR mutation), Shwachman-Diamond Syndrome, Alagille's syndrome (JAG1 gene), and others. There's a strong chance you'll be asked at least one question about a genetic disorder, so learn these well before the test.

- **To ERCP, or not to ERCP?** That is the question. Not only is this crucial to understand in clinical practice, but Board examiners want to know that you won't do an ERCP at the drop of a hat and that you understand whether and when it's an appropriate test. For example, if you have a strong pretest likelihood of a retained duct stone in acute cholecystitis, then ERCP is warranted. But if you have a low or medium pretest likelihood, then it's probably not appropriate. Or, you might get a case of pancreas divisum in an asymptomatic person— don't think about doing ERCP there because divisum occurs in 7% of the population and is not thought to cause pancreatitis in everyone. Or maybe you'll get a case of functional GI pain that mimics sphincter of Oddi spasm but is not associated with any abnormal tests or imaging. Again, don't do an ERCP there (please)! The overarching theme is to be careful when you order (or do) an ERCP; we've come up with a variety of cases that will test your trigger finger. The malpractice attorneys also do not want to see trigger-happy interventional endoscopists!

- **Gallstones.** Gallstones are a dime a dozen, so it makes sense they'll show up on your Board exam in one way or another. Know the 3 major types of gallstones (black pigment, brown pigment, cholesterol) and in which conditions they occur. For example, if we were to ask you which type of stone is seen in recurrent pyogenic cholangitis, what would you say? How about in cirrhosis? What about in neurofibromatosis? Stay tuned, we have answers later in the book. Also know how to recognize gallstones that stray off the beaten path, like a stone in the stomach via cholegastro fistula (Bouveret's syndrome), a gallbladder infundibulum or cystic duct stone compressing the common hepatic duct (Mirizzi's syndrome), or a stone jammed in the ileocecal valve with concurrent pneumobilia and dilated loops of small bowel (Rigler's triad). All classics, and all in the book.

- **Iatrogenica imperfecta.** Yep, doctors make mistakes and are sometimes imperfect. This is especially true in ERCP and laparoscopic cholecystectomy, procedures that are safe but high volume, so it's just a matter of time before you come across complications. Be ready to recognize a retroperitoneal vs lateral duodenal wall perforation from ERCP. Know when to worry about an air embolism in a patient decompensating during a procedure. Memorize all the risk factors (and there are a lot of them) for post-ERCP pancreatitis, and know how to reduce the risk of this common and morbid condition. After a cholecystectomy, be ready to identify and manage a biloma, bile duct transection, stump leak, and retained surgical clip. Similarly, know the biliary complications of liver transplant, including bile duct stricture, anastomotic leaks, ischemic cholangitis, and fibrosing cholestatic hepatitis from HCV.

- **Pancreatic cancer.** Pancreatic cancer remains a devastating and all-too-common disease. As of the writing of this book, we still have very few effective therapies for pancreatic cancer other than early detection and surgical resection, which itself can still be unsuccessful. Know that when a middle-aged person has a pancreatic head mass, you should proceed quickly to surgery unless there are contraindications. Know the main contraindications to surgery, including high comorbidities, involvement of the great vessels, and metastatic spread. Don't be fooled into doing a bunch of preoperative evaluations, like ERCP with brushings (often not helpful), EUS, and so forth—go to surgery. We cover this in depth later in the book. For patients with unresectable disease, know when to place a palliative stent and whether to use a plastic stent vs self-expanding metallic stent (SEMS).

- **Pancreatic neuroendocrine tumors (PNETs).** PNETs are rare in real life, but very common in Board review. These tumors are highly testable because they present with characteristic syndromes that features all sorts of classic Board buzzwords. For example, what PNET is associated with neurofibromatosois and causes gallstones? What PNET is associated with rhabdomyoma, angiomyolipoma, and tuberous sclerosis? What PNET causes profound hypochlorhydria, and why? Which is associated with migratory necrolytic necrosis? We include a table of PNET associations and buzzwords, and cover individual PNETs in a variety of vignettes later in the book.

- **Drug-induced pancreatitis.** In the liver *Acing* book we covered drug-induced liver disease (DILI) in great depth because Board examiners want to make sure you can recognize potentially reversible, iatrogenic damage. In this book, we cover a range of drug-induced pancreatitis scenarios. Know the most common, so-called "Class 1" agents strongly tied to pancreatitis. Be ready to recognize drug-induced pancreatitis in an inflammatory bowel disease patient taking azathioprine, mesalamine, or steroids. What if an FAP patient develops pancreatitis? There are nondrug reasons for pancreatitis in FAP (Can you think of one?), but also drug-induced pancreatitis (What medicine are we thinking of here?). What antisecretory medication is associated with pancreatitis? Which antihypertensives and antiarrhytmics? All fair game.

So, those are the panc-bil highlights that could appear on the Boards. Of course, there are many other important panc-bil topics that might show up on the test, and we've done our best to create a single volume that captures the classics. Keep in mind that this volume is not meant to be all-inclusive. We also cover many panc-bil topics elsewhere in the *Acing* series, so this book is best read alongside the other volumes. Nonetheless, these vignettes should be quite helpful in daily practice as we review so many important clinical scenarios that you are bound to encounter in the clinical trenches.

One thing you don't need to know, however, are the very technical details of advanced endoscopic techniques. The Board exam is not a test specifically for interventional endoscopists alone, but rather for general gastroenterologists. For example, you may need to decide whether to place a plastic stent vs SEMS for a malignant biliary obstruction, but not necessarily for procedural details about how to place the stent. Similarly, it is important to understand when to perform endoscopic vs surgical necrosectomy of nonviable pancreatic tissue, but not crucial to diagram the step by step technical details of these procedures. Bottom line: know whether and when advanced procedures are warranted, but not necessarily how to technically perform the procedures.

That's it for now. Let's get this thing started.

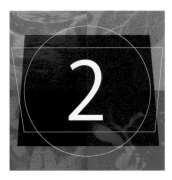

"TOUGH STUFF" VIGNETTES

In the pages that follow are 73 "tough stuff" vignettes. As described in the Preface, these have been culled from years of clinical practice experience and teaching Board review. They have also been iteratively reviewed and vetted with our GI fellows at Cedars-Sinai Medical Center and our colleagues at Atlanta Gastroenterology Associates and Emory University. In addition, we offer an annual live, in-person *Acing the GI Board Exam* review course where we continuously refine, update, and perfect our vignettes and "Here's the Point!" learning pearls. We've written this book in the style of our courses; the in-person course is a good opportunity to reinforce the vignettes you'll read here and in the other *Acing* volumes. You can also access additional questions in a different multiple-choice format online in the *Acing the GI Board Exam* question bank (www.acingboardexams.com).

As you go through these vignettes, keep the following points in mind:

- These are generally difficult. That is by design. You may still know the answers to many of these vignettes—a sign that you are well prepared for the exam. But if you can't get them all right, that's fine too. That's the whole point of this book—to ensure that you are gaining incremental information, not just reviewing stuff you already know. Keep in mind, however, that for every tough question that's in this book, there are a bunch of gimmies that don't appear in this book. The entire Board exam won't be full of "tough stuff" questions. Don't get too demoralized if you can't correctly answer all of these questions. Rest assured that you already know most of the gimmies just by paying attention and learning during your clinical experiences.

- These are in completely random order—there's no explicit rhyme or reason. See the Preface for our rationale of using a random order.

Spiegel BMR, Karsan HA.
Acing the Pancreaticobiliary Questions on the GI Board Exam:
The Ultimate Crunch-Time Resource (pp 5-136).
© 2018 Taylor & Francis Group.

- The vignettes appear on one page, followed by one or more open-ended questions. The answers are provided on the next page. Before you turn the page, take a moment to really think about the answers. Even if you're not sure of the answer, at least take a moment to think about the potential differential diagnosis, or other information you might need to better answer the question. This form of active learning is more useful than merely flipping the page and reading the answer. Seriously… don't just flip the page until you've given the vignette at least a nanosecond of thought. The answer will be more meaningful if you've first struggled a bit to think through the vignette.

- After each answer, there is a short section entitled "Why Might This Be Tested?" The purpose of this entry is to emphasize why it's important to know the content of each vignette, vis à vis for Board review in particular. It puts you in the mindset of why certain topics are important to better understand their potential reasoning, and might help you better remember each vignette.

- At the bottom of each answer page there is a box entitled: "Here's the Point!" This is meant to summarize the key issue or issues that appear on the page. If you're really in crunch time, then you should, at the very least, make sure you know the "Here's the Point!" bottom line for each vignette. The "Crunch-Time" Self-Test on page 139 catalogues all of these facts (and more) into one 150-question test, and quizzes you to see if you can remember the key points from each vignette. Some of the answer pages also have a "Clinical Threshold Alert," followed by the presentation of an explicit clinical threshold (see the Preface for details).

Vignette 1: All in the FAMMMily

A 50-year-old woman presents with 2 months of weight loss without abdominal pain. Three weeks ago, she noticed dark urine, clay-colored stools, and yellowing of her eyes and skin. She has been experiencing fatigue and itching over the last 2 weeks. She has previously been healthy. She has never consumed alcohol, smoked cigarrettes, or used any illicit drugs. Her family history is significant for multiple first and second degree family members with melanoma and pancreatic cancer. Vital signs are temperature 98.4°F, blood pressure 120/80 mm Hg, heart rate 90 beats/minute, and oxygen saturation 100% on room air. On physical exam, there is scleral and cutaneous icterus. Her abdomen is soft and not tender. There are multiple nevi throughout her body (below in Figure 1-1). Liver tests show total bilirubin 6 mg/dL, alkaline phosphatase 405 U/L, AST 101 U/L, and ALT 115 U/L. A CT scan is obtained and demonstrates a 3.5-cm heterogeneous mass in the head of the pancreas. EUS with fine needle aspiration (FNA) is performed. Cytology is consistent with pancreatic adenocarcinoma.

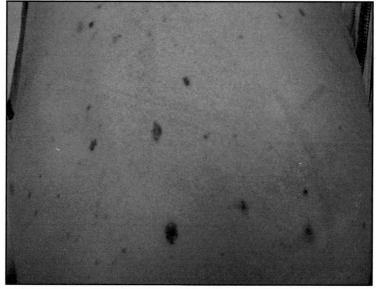

Figure 1-1. Several dysplastic nevi on back. (Reprinted with permission from Jamie B. MacKelfresh, MD, Emory University.)

▶ *Why did this patient develop pancreatic adenocarcinoma?*

Vignette 1: Answer

Yes, the title gives this one away; we decided to start by throwing a softball. This patient has FAMMM syndrome (familial atypical multiple mole melanoma syndrome). This rare syndrome occurs due to autosomal dominant mutations in CDKN2A, a tumor suppressor gene located on chromosome 9. Patients with FAMMM syndrome have multiple nevi, cutaneous and ocular melanomas, and an increased risk of pancreatic cancer. The cumulative risk of pancreatic cancer in these patients is as high as 17% by age 75. As an aside, don't say malignant melanoma. That is redundant. All melanomas are malignant. You don't say "benign adenoma," right? So, it is just melanoma. Anyway…

Genetic causes of pancreatic cancer are uncommon in clinical practice, but important for Board review. You should therefore commit to memory the most well documented genetic risk factors for pancreatic cancer (Table 1-1)—this stuff is absolute gold for Board preparation. Know the autosomal dominant PRSS-1 mutation (which we will discuss soon), and autosomal recessive SPINK1 mutations. BRCA mutations are best known for their tendency to increase breast cancer risk, but you should know that they also increase the risk of pancreatic adenocarcinoma, particularly the BRCA2 mutations. STK11 mutations are inherited in an autosomal dominant fashion and are particularly high yield, since they cause the Peutz-Jeghers syndrome of hamartomatous polyps throughout the GI tract and hyperpigmented macules on the lips and oral mucosa. The polyps in Peutz-Jeghers syndrome don't generally develop into cancer, but they can grow to large sizes and cause bowel obstruction, particularly in the small intestine. Peutz-Jeghers syndrome predisposes to many cancers in the GI tract and reproductive organs. The lifetime risk for any malignancy is as high as 85%, and the risk of pancreatic cancer is about 10% to 15% in patients with Peutz-Jeghers syndrome.

Lynch syndrome results from mutations in mismatch repair genes, particularly MSH1, MSH2, MSH6, and PMS2. This syndrome is also very important for Board review due to its association with colorectal cancer (see original *Acing* book for more). It's worth remembering the other Lynch-related cancers, one of which is pancreatic adenocarcinoma.

Table 1-1. GENETIC SYNDROMES WITH INCREASED PANCREATIC CANCER RISK. THIS TABLE IS **SOLID GOLD.** KNOW THE WHOLE THING!		
Syndrome	Gene Mutation	Other Cancers
Autosomal dominant hereditary pancreatitis	PRSS-1	
Autosomal recessive hereditary pancreatitis	SPINK1	
Peutz-Jeghers syndrome	STK11 (also called LKB1)	• GI: Esophagus, stomach, small intestine, colorectal, and gallbladder cancer • GU: Breast, ovarian, cervical cancer, and testicular cancer • Lung cancer
FAMMM syndrome	CDKN2A	• Melanoma
Lynch syndrome	DNA mismatch repair genes	• Colorectal cancer • Endometrial cancer • Visceral carcinomas • Gliomas • Cutaneous keratoacanthomas and sebaceous tumors
Hereditary breast cancer	BRCA2	• Breast cancer • Ovarian cancer • Prostate cancer

Here's the Point!

Family history of melanoma + Family history of pancreatic cancer + Multiple nevi = FAMMM syndrome

Vignette 2: A PReSSing Problem

A 20-year-old man has chronic, constant epigastric pain radiating to the back. He has a history of recurrent acute pancreatitis during his teenage years. He has 2 siblings. His sister has had a similar clinical course, while his brother has no symptoms. His father and paternal grandfather had chronic pancreatitis and died of pancreatic cancer in their 50s and 60s respectively. He recently started to smoke cigarrettes but denies any alcohol or illicit drug use. On CT scan, there is pancreatic duct dilation and parenchymal calcifications. He undergoes endoscopic ultrasound which does not detect any pancreatic mass but does reveal pancreatic duct dilation, calcifications, lobularity, and hyperechoic strands.

▶ *What is the cause of this patient's symptoms?*

▶ *What can he do to reduce his risk of pancreatic cancer?*

Vignette 2: Answer

The patient has autosomal dominant hereditary pancreatitis. This disorder occurs due to mutations in the serine protease-1 gene (PRSS-1). The PRSS-1 gene encodes a cationic trypsinogen called trypsin-1. Mutations in PRSS-1 lead to excessive trypsin. Excessive trypsin causes premature activation of pancreatic digestive enzymes and pancreatic injury. Patients with hereditary pancreatitis typically present with recurrent acute pancreatitis in childhood and adolescence, and chronic pancreatitis in late adolescence or early adulthood.

Hereditary pancreatitis markedly increases the risk of pancreatic cancer after the age of 50 years. Smoking doubles the risk of pancreatic cancer in these patients, so you must recommend smoking cessation. Islet cell transplantation and pancreatectomy have been offered as options but their use is controversial, which means that it's not really important for Board review. Pancreatic cancer screening with cross-sectional imaging and/or endoscopic ultrasound is frequently offered to patients with hereditary pancreatitis and other genetic conditions that predispose to pancreatic adenocarcinoma. But that isn't evidence-based either without clear mortality benefit. Bottom line: know PRSS-1 and its clinical association.

Why Might This Be Tested? Genetics are classic Board review fodder, particularly when a well-defined genetic mutation leads to a common gastroenterologic condition.

Here's the Point!

> **Young adult + Chronic pancreatitis + Multiple family members with pancreatic cancer = PRSS-1 gene mutation**

Vignette 3: Pancreatic Insufficiency and Colonic Obstruction

An 18-year-old Caucasian male presents to the emergency department with acute onset of diffuse abdominal pain. He has a longstanding history of chronic diarrhea for which he takes high doses of pancreatic enzyme supplements. He has had several episodes of pneumonia throughout his life, and has chronic sinusitis. He does not smoke cigarettes or drink any alcohol. Vital signs are temperature 100.1°F, blood pressure 95/65 mm Hg, and heart rate 111 beats/minute. Oxygen saturation is at his baseline of 90% on 2 L. On physical exam, there is diffuse tenderness to palpation. White blood cell (WBC) count is 11.2K, and fecal elastase is 40 mcg/g. Abdominal X-ray reveals dilated small bowel loops with a transition point in the left colon, and decompressed bowel distal to the transition point. A nasogastric and a rectal tube is placed upon admission to the hospital. Despite 48 hours of conservative management, his symptoms do not improve so he undergoes a left hemicolectomy. Pathology demonstrates submucosal fibrosis and stenosis of the colon.

► *Why does the patient have pancreatic insufficiency?*

► *What caused the colonic obstruction?*

Vignette 3: Answer

This patient has cystic fibrosis. This autosomal recessive condition results from mutations in the cystic fibrosis transmembrane conductance regulator (CFTR) gene. The CFTR gene encodes a chloride channel protein. Defective chloride transport caused by this mutation results in thick, viscous secretions in the lungs, pancreas and other organs. In the pancreas, the thick secretions cause pancreatic duct obstruction, and progressive parenchymal damage. Clinically significant pancreatic insufficiency occurs in most patients with cystic fibrosis. With the adoption of universal newborn screening in the United States, most patients with cystic fibrosis are diagnosed in infancy. If you suspect undiagnosed cystic fibrosis, the initial evaluation is to order a sweat chloride test. A level ≥ 60 mmol/L is considered abnormal. The diagnosis can then be confirmed with DNA testing.

Of note, a different form of hereditary pancreatitis, involving the SPINK1 (Serine Protease INhibitor Kazal type 1 gene) can also be inherited in an autosomal recessive fashion. This can also cause chronic pancreatitis and pancreatic insufficiency. However, cystic fibrosis is much more likely in this patient with pneumonia and sinusitis.

Patients taking high doses of pancreatic enzyme supplements over a prolonged period can develop fibrosing colonopathy. In these patients, histology reveals characteristic submucosal fibrosis that results in colonic strictures and stenosis. The exact pathogenesis of this rare condition is unknown, and we don't know if lowering the lipase dose leads to regression of fibrosis. But we do know overloading on enzymes can do some major damage—like what happened here. In general, the lipase dose should not exceed 10,000 units/kg/day or 2500 units/kg of body weight/meal.

Why Might This Be Tested? This is a classic pediatric GI condition that you will encounter more often in the adult realm as the life expectancy has risen for these patients over time. This multi-system illness has important GI manifestations and a well-established genetic defect.

Clinical Threshold Alert 1: Fecal elastase < 200 mcg/g suggests pancreatic exocrine insufficiency; fecal elastase < 100 mcg/g indicates severe pancreatic exocrine insufficiency.

Clinical Threshold Alert 2: Sweat chloride is typically ≥ 60 mmol/L in cystic fibrosis.

Clinical Threshold Alert 3: Supplemental lipase dose should not exceed 10,000 units/kg/day or 2500 units/kg of body weight/meal.

Here's the Point! 1

**Chronic pancreatitis + Autosomal recessive inheritance =
CFTR mutation (cystic fibrosis) or SPINK1 mutation**

Here's the Point! 2

**High doses of pancreatic enzyme supplements + Colonic stricture =
Fibrosing colonopathy**

Vignette 4: Pregnant With Pancreatitis

A 27-year-old woman in her third trimester of pregnancy presents with acute onset of epigastric pain radiating to the back along with nausea and vomiting. In addition to epigastric tenderness to palpation, physical examination demonstrates the following lesions on the extensor surfaces of her arms shown below in Figure 4-1. Her blood pressure is 106/62 mm Hg, and heart rate is 112 beats/minute. Serum lipase level is 5600 U/L, urine pregnancy test is positive and ketones are normal. Serum lactate is 5 mmol/L, serum creatinine is 2.3 mg/dL, serum calcium is 6 mg/dL, and blood glucose level is 110 mg/dL. She does not drink any alcohol. Her only medication is prenatal vitamins. Right upper quadrant ultrasound does not demonstrate any stones or sludge. Her family history is significant only for early cardiovascular disease.

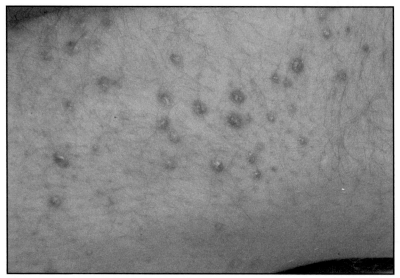

Figure 4-1. Lesions on extensor surfaces of arms. (Reprinted with permission from Robert A. Swerlick, MD, Emory University.)

▶ *In addition to aggressive fluid resuscitation and analgesia, what additional therapy could you recommend in the acute setting?*

Vignette 4: Answer

This patient most likely has hypertriglyceridemia-induced pancreatitis. Hypertriglyceridemia is the third most common cause of acute pancreatitis after alcohol and gallstones. This vignette excludes alcohol and gallstones, so based on statistical likelihood alone you could guess hypertriglyceridemia as the etiology and have a good chance of being correct. This patient also has eruptive xanthomas, a characteristic finding of hypertriglyceridemia, from deposition of cholesterol-rich material forming yellow and red papules. Remember that skin manifestations of GI and liver diseases are important for Board review; this is another in a long line of dermatology examples covered in this and the other *Acing* books.

By the way, random question: What skin lesion is found in glucagonoma? We'll cover it later. Also, what skin lesion is found on the elbows in celiac disease? And how does celiac disease affect the pancreas? More on that later, too.

Back to hypertriglyceridemia. When triglyceride levels exceed > 1000 mg/dL the risk of pancreatitis begins to rise significantly. That's a good threshold to remember. At this level, breakdown of triglycerides by lipases to toxic free fatty acids can lead to lipotoxicity and pancreatitis. The patient in this vignette is pregnant. That's relevant, because pregnancy increases triglyceride levels particularly in the third trimester, and 50% to 60% of acute pancreatitis occurring during pregnancy is attributed to hypertriglyceridemia. Triglyceride levels typically only rise to about 300 mg/dL during pregnancy, so a predisposing inherited condition is likely in this case. Among the familial dyslipidemias, type IV (high levels of very low-density lipoprotein) usually requires another factor to raise serum triglyceride levels (like pregnancy). Unlike other familial dyslipidemias, type IV tends to present in adulthood. The patient in this vignette likely has type IV familial dyslipidemia, which is inherited in an autosomal dominant fashion.

Since we're on the topic of conditions that increase triglyceride levels, you should also remember other common predisposing factors: diabetic ketoacidosis (suspect if the patient has a low pH and high ketones), hypothyroidism, and estrogen replacement or tamoxifen.

It's important to initiate aggressive intravenous hydration for every patient with acute pancreatitis. In fact, data indicate that hydration is most beneficial during the first 12 to 24 hours of management, and may have less benefit beyond this initial period (not that you should stop giving intravenous fluids, but always be sure to start right away). In addition to managing pain with appropriate analgesics, you might initiate therapeutic plasma exchange in this patient with hypertriglyceridemia-induced pancreatitis who also has a lipase level > 3 times the upper limit of normal, hypocalcemia, lactic acidosis, and signs of organ dysfunction. If the patient's blood sugar were higher than 500 mg/dL, then intravenous insulin may also be beneficial. Insulin enhances lipoprotein lipase and accelerates chylomicron and VLDL metabolism—both helpful when your body is swimming in triglycerides. While oral lipid lowering drugs like gemfibrozil are indicated in the long term to maintain low triglyceride levels, they are unlikely to be tolerated or work quickly enough to help in the acute setting.

Why Might This Be Tested? Hypertriglyceridemia-induced pancreatitis is the third most common cause of pancreatitis, so you are likely to encounter this condition a few times during your career. Plus, you gotta know your derm manifestations of GI and liver diseases, and this is another classic.

Clinical Threshold Alert: Hypertriglyceridemia is considered a risk for pancreatitis when levels are > 1000 mg/dL. Consider therapeutic plasma exchange for acute pancreatitis when serum triglycerides > 1000 mg/dL, lipase > 3 times the upper limit of normal, hypocalcemia, lactic acidosis, and signs of organ dysfunction are present. Initiate intravenous insulin for hypertriglyceridemia induced pancreatitis when serum glucose > 500 mg/dL.

Here's the Point! 1

Acute pancreatitis + Xanthomas + Predisposing condition (pregnancy, diabetes, hypothyroidism, or estrogen replacement) = Think hypertriglyceridemia-induced pancreatitis

Here's the Point! 2

Unlike other familial dyslipidemias, type IV tends to present in adulthood.

Vignettes 5-9: Take a DIP

A PubMed search makes it seem like virtually any medication can cause acute pancreatitis. Unlike drug induced liver injury, or DILI (see the hepatology book in the *Acing* series for more on that), there are no distinguishing laboratory or pathologic features in drug-induced pancreatitis (DIP). You clearly do not need to know every medication that has been reported to cause pancreatitis—that would be a maddening feat of memorization. But there is a group of commonly used medications where the data strongly support a link to acute pancreatitis; these are called "Class I" drugs.

For completeness, Class I comes in 2 types, Class Ia and Class Ib. Class Ia drugs are known to cause acute pancreatitis upon rechallenge in the absence of other potential etiologies. Class Ib drugs are similar, but published case reports were not able to completely exclude other causes of pancreatitis during rechallenge. Class II through Class IV drugs have increasingly less evidence of causation—the exact criteria are not worth memorizing for Board review.

In any event, you should be able to identify the Class I agent both in clinical practice and on the Boards. For each of the vignettes below, identify the most likely Class I medication to have caused acute pancreatitis. Assume that other causes of acute pancreatitis have already been ruled out.

5. Three weeks after initiating an oral medication for moderately severe Crohn's disease, a patient develops acute pancreatitis. He was told he needs to monitor his blood counts every few weeks after initiating the drug.

6. A patient with familial adenomatous polyposis has 2 episodes of acute pancreatitis. For about a year, he has been taking a medication to reduce risk of adenoma formation. He has a history of proctocolectomy and ileoanal pouch anastomosis for early stage colon adenocarcinoma and polyps with high-grade dysplasia.

7. Four months after initiating an anticonvulsant to reduce risk of seizures, a patient develops severe acute pancreatitis requiring admission to the intensive care unit.

8. An otherwise healthy 20-year-old man presents with an episode of acute pancreatitis. On physical examination, there is bilateral gynecomastia. He denies taking any medications.

9. A 34-year-old woman develops acute pancreatitis 10 weeks after starting an antibiotic for a urinary tract infection.

Vignettes 5-9: Answers

5.   This is pancreatitis due to azathioprine (AZA) or 6-mercaptopurine (6-MP). AZA or 6-MP induced pancreatitis is immunologically mediated, and therefore tends to occur 1 to 6 weeks after initiation, and 1 to 3 days after a rechallenge. The reported incidence of AZA/6-MP-induced pancreatitis is 2% to 6%, so it's not all that uncommon. Mesalamine is another inflammatory bowel disease (IBD) medication that can cause acute immunologically mediated acute pancreatitis and requires monitoring of blood counts. However, this drug is not routinely recommended in patients with Crohn's disease due to lack of significant efficacy. If the patient in the vignette had ulcerative colitis, then either mesalamine or AZA/6-MP would have been possible etiologies. Timing of drug initiation would be the best way to discern between these medications that can cause acute pancreatitis. Steroids can also cause acute pancreatitis, but do not require routine monitoring of blood counts. See the IBD *Acing* book for more on these drugs.

Why Might This Be Tested? AZA/6-MP induced pancreatitis is high yield for Board review, since it ties together 2 major disease conditions in gastroenterology (IBD and acute pancreatitis).

Here's the Point!

> **IBD + Acute pancreatitis = Could be from mesalamine, AZA/6-MP, or steroids**

6.   Sulindac is the most likely offending medication. This nonsteroidal is not routinely recommended to reduce adenoma risk in all patients with familial adenomatous polyposis (FAP). However, in patients with FAP who have had colectomy with ileoanal anastomosis, sulindac may reduce the size and number of adenomatous polyps. The latency from initiation of the drug to onset of acute pancreatitis ranges anywhere from a month to several years, so it's important not to ignore sulindac as a potential etiology of pancreatitis even if it was not recently initiated.

Why Might This Be Tested? This is a classic example of a "twofer"—you know, "two for the price of one." In this case, the twofer question ties together 2 major topics in gastroenterology—acute pancreatitis and colon cancer prevention in familial adenomatous polyposis.

Here's the Point!

> **FAP patient with history of colectomy + Acute pancreatitis = Think sulindac**

7.   This is probably a consequence of valproic acid. Valproic acid is funny—it's a medicine you probably can't remember ever prescribing, much less recently, but the side effect profile is very important to understand. Just know valproic acid (it comes up in other *Acing* books in this series). Pancreatitis from valproic acid results from accumulation of a toxic metabolite, so latency from initiation to development of pancreatitis is typically 3 to 6 months, and rechallenge latency is 1.5 to 3 months. Prompt discontinuation is important because valproic acid tends to cause severe pancreatitis, with complications such as necrosis, pseudocyst, and even death has been reported. By the way, what else does valproic acid do of relevance to GI Board review? Sit on that one for a second. We'll come back to it soon. But really, think about it… how could valproic acid show up in a multiple-choice question? Stay tuned.

Why Might This Be Tested? Because the side effect profile of valproic acid is extremely important.

Here's the Point!

Seizures or bipolar disorder + Severe acute pancreatitis = Consider valproic acid

8.   This is a trick question, since the patient is not taking any medications. However, the physical finding of bilateral gynecomastia should raise suspicion for marijuana use. This patient has cannabis-induced pancreatitis, due to inhaled marijuana. Cannabis is the most popular illicit drug in the United States, so its association with acute pancreatitis is a very reasonable topic for Board review. While we're on this topic, what other GI conditions are associated with cannabis use? Right. Cyclical vomiting syndrome (CVS) and cannabis hyperemesis syndrome (CHS). You should know about these, too, and they're covered in other *Acing* editions. Oh, by the way, what else can cause gynecomastia and pancreatitis other than cannabis? We can think of 3 other things.

Why Might This Be Tested? Because there is plenty of cannabis involved in Board review (…or at least, discussing the side effects of cannabis use). ☺

Here's the Point!

Gynecomastia + Acute pancreatitis = Think of inhaled marijuana

9.   The patient has sulfonamide-induced pancreatitis, likely due to trimethoprim-sulfa-methoxazole (TMP-SMX). The latency period is typically 10 weeks. TMP-SMX is yet another Board review favorite. What other bad thing does TMP-SMX do that is important for GI Board review? And what classic GI condition can TMP-SMX treat?

Why Might This Be Tested? Because TMP-SMX sounds like a bad mid-1980s cover band.

Here's the Point!

Urinary tract infection + Antibiotic + Acute pancreatitis = TMP-SMX

In the first *Acing* book we provide a memory aid to help you organize the various medications associated with pancreatitis. Here it is, below in Figure 9-1, so you don't need to flip back and forth between books. Below that is a more conventional table of Class I agent associations with acute pancreatitis in Table 9-1.

```
        P entamidine
        A zathioprine
        N
        C imetidine
  valp R oic acid
        E strogens
    5 - A SA
        T etracycline
    Dd  I
    HC  T Z
        I
    La  S ix-MP; Salicylates; Sulfonamides
```

Figure 9-1. Memory aid to recall medications associated with pancreatitis.

Table 9-1.
DRUGS WITH A CLASS 1* ASSOCIATION WITH ACUTE PANCREATITIS

- Antiarrhythmics: Amiodarone, Procainamide
- Anticonvulsants: Valproic Acid
- Antihypertensives: Enalapril, Losartan, Furosemide
- Antimicrobials: Isoniazid, Dapsone, Metronidazole, Pentamidine, Sulfa drugs, Tetracycline
- Antivirals: Lamivudine, Nelfinavir
- IBD medications: Azothioprine, 6-MP, mesalamine, and steroids
- Chemotherapeutic agents: All-trans-retinoic acid, ifosfamide
- Illicit drugs: Cannabis (inhaled)
- Statins: Pravastatin, Simvastatin
- Other: Methimazole, Sulindac

*At least one case report describes a recurrence of acute pancreatitis with drug rechallenge.

Oh, right, we almost forgot. What else does valproic acid do? It can cause microvesicular steatosis of the liver. Know that. And what else can TMP-SMX do that's bad? It can cause an acute cholestatic injury biochemically marked by an alkaline phosphatase (ALP) level twice the upper limit of normal and an ALT/ALP ratio < 2. What GI conditions can TMP-SMX treat? It's used for Whipple's Disease and Isospora (see the first *Acing* book for more). Plus other stuff, but know those 2 for sure. Finally, what else beyond cannabis causes both gynecomastia and pancreatitis? Cimetidine, anabolic steroids, and alcoholism.

Vignette 10: More Skin Stuff (and Pancreatitis)

A 25-year-old South Asian woman is admitted with her second episode of acute pancreatitis. She has a longstanding history of abdominal bloating and diarrhea, primarily in the summertime. However, once she moved to the United States a year ago her symptoms have persisted. She does not drink any alcohol. She does smoke a half pack of cigarettes a day. She does not have a family history of pancreatitis or pancreatic cancer but does have a family history of type 1 diabetes. She is scheduled to see a dermatologist to evaluate an intensely itchy rash she developed several weeks ago. On physical exam, there is a papulovesicular rash on her elbows and knees. Her laboratory studies are significant for hemoglobin 9.8 g/dL, MCV 75, serum ferritin 5 ng/mL, normal WBC count, platelet count, normal serum calcium, normal liver enzymes, and normal triglycerides. Her right upper quadrant ultrasound is normal. Serum ANA and IgG4 are normal. An MRI is obtained, and reveals normal pancreatic duct size and anatomy. No pancreatic mass lesion, bile duct dilation, or bile duct stones are identified.

▶ *What is the most likely cause of this patient's pancreatitis?*

▶ *What additional tests are warranted?*

▶ *What measures should you recommend to reduce the risk of recurrent pancreatitis?*

Vignette 10: Answer

This patient's recurrent episodes of acute pancreatitis are most likely due to celiac disease. Duodenal inflammation from celiac disease can cause papillary stenosis and obstruction of pancreatic duct outflow, resulting in acute pancreatitis. The clues provided in this vignette are chronic diarrhea, iron deficiency anemia due to iron malabsorption, and the pathognomonic dermatitis herpetiformis rash. Elevated serum tissue transglutaminase and duodenal biopsies should establish the diagnosis. This patient should also undergo upper endoscopy with a side-viewing duodenoscope to rule out an ampullary mass or a periampullary diverticulum, and an endoscopic ultrasound to evaluate for an occult pancreatic malignancy.

Notice that the patient in this vignette was not of northern European origin. An increasing prevalence of celiac disease is being recognized in many other parts of the world. Northern India is a region with a relatively high prevalence of celiac disease. Patients in this region typically experience a "summer diarrhea" because wheat is traditionally consumed in the summer months, and bread made from maize is consumed during the remainder of the year. Interesting, isn't it?

So, will a gluten-free diet for this patient lead to resolution of duodenal inflammation and papillary outflow obstruction? Yes, it can. Powerful stuff. Also, since smoking is an independent risk factor for acute pancreatitis, you should strongly advise her to quit smoking in addition to initiating a gluten-free diet.

Why Might This Be Tested? Because it seems like celiac disease can do anything. In addition to causing epilepsy through occipital calcifications, presenting with Howell-Jolly body anemia, and mimicking IBS (important for Board review), celiac can also cause acute pancreatitis—another rare but testable association. We cover the other associations elsewhere in the *Acing* series.

Here's the Point!

> **Chronic diarrhea + Iron deficiency anemia + Unexplained recurrent Acute pancreatitis = Think of celiac disease**

Vignette 11: Double Trouble

A 71-year-old male is seen in consultation because he has had 3 episodes of acute pancreatitis in the last 6 months. He is currently asymptomatic. He has not experienced any unintentional weight loss. He does not take any medications and has never consumed alcohol. There is no history of abdominal trauma. Vital signs are temperature 98.5°F, blood pressure 121/85 mm Hg, pulse 80 beats/minute, and oxygen saturation 98% on room air. On examination, he appears to be comfortable. There is no abdominal tenderness to palpation. Complete blood count, serum chemistry, liver tests, serum calcium, triglyceride, ANA and IgG4 are normal. A right upper quadrant ultrasound is obtained and does not demonstrate any gallstones. His last screening colonoscopy was 1 year ago and was normal. On MRI, his common bile duct is dilated to 10 mm with smooth distal tapering and his pancreatic duct is dilated to 5 mm with smooth distal tapering. He undergoes duodenoscopy and endoscopic ultrasound, which does not reveal an occult pancreatic malignancy but does reveal the finding in Figure 11-1.

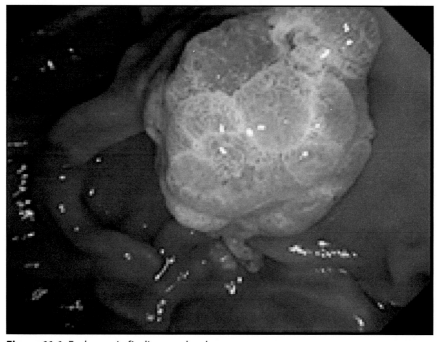

Figure 11-1. Endoscopic finding on duodenoscopy.

▶ *What is this finding?*

▶ *How should you manage this finding?*

Vignette 11: Answer

This patient has an ampullary adenoma, which can cause recurrent acute pancreatitis due to pancreatic outflow obstruction. Ampullary adenomas occur commonly in patients with familial adenomatous polyposis (FAP), but they can also occur sporadically. Ampullary adenomas that occur in the setting of FAP tend to have a lower risk of progressing to carcinoma than sporadic adenomas. Nevertheless, options for managing any asymptomatic ampullary adenoma are resection vs ongoing surveillance. Ongoing surveillance is reasonable if there are no foci of high-grade dysplasia and no extension of the tumor into the bile duct or pancreatic duct. If a surveillance strategy is selected, there is not a clear consensus as to the exact interval, which means surveillance strategies don't need to be discussed further for Board review.

This patient has a symptomatic sporadic ampullary adenoma that requires removal. Endoscopic ampullectomy is an option for patients with adenomas < 2 to 3 cm, no lymph nodes on preprocedure imaging, and no extension of the tumor into the bile duct or pancreatic duct on endoscopic ultrasound. This patient successfully underwent an endoscopic ampullectomy, and had no evidence of recurrent adenoma on postprocedure surveillance duodenoscopy. Endoscopic ampullectomy poses a high risk of postprocedure pancreatitis, so pancreatic stenting and rectal indomethacin is recommended, but more on that in a later vignette. After endoscopic ampullectomy, a surveillance duodenoscopy is recommended after 1 to 6 months, and then every 3 to 12 months for 2 years.

Know that in general, surgical options are a pancreaticoduodenectomy (Whipple procedure) vs a surgical ampullectomy. The recurrence rates are much higher after a surgical ampullectomy, but morbidity is higher with a Whipple resection.

Why Might This Be Tested? A dilated bile duct and pancreatic duct (ie "double duct sign") always raises the possibility of an occult pancreatic malignancy, but outflow obstruction from an ampullary adenoma can also cause these findings. Remember, that the "double duct sign" is "double trouble"—it's never good. It is also important to recognize the possibilities. That is, when a patient presents with an unexplained double duct sign, you should evaluate the ampulla with a side-viewing duodenoscope and perform an endoscopic ultrasound to assess for an occult pancreatic malignancy.

Clinical Threshold Alert: So long as an ampullary adenoma is < 2 to 3 cm in size, and assuming there are no lymph nodes on imaging or extension of the tumor into the ductal systems on EUS, endoscopic ampullectomy remains a treatment option.

Here's the Point! 1

Idiopathic recurrent acute pancreatitis = Perform EUS to assess for occult pancreatic malignancy

Here's the Point! 2

Idiopathic recurrent acute pancreatitis + Pancreatic or bile duct dilation = Perform EUS + Side-viewing examination to rule out ampullary adenoma or periampullary diverticulum

Vignette 12: Perfect Storm

A 27-year-old woman undergoes an ERCP for suspected biliary sphincter of Oddi dysfunction. She underwent a cholecystectomy for symptomatic cholelithiasis 3 years ago. Her symptoms initially resolved, but approximately 1 year ago she began experiencing episodes of right upper quadrant pain. Her AST and ALT increases to 150 and 250 U/L during episodes, but are normal in between episodes. An MRI did not reveal any bile duct stones, pancreatic or biliary duct dilation. Prior to the procedure, her physical examination was unremarkable, with no abdominal tenderness to palpation. Biliary cannulation proves to be difficult. The pancreatic duct is cannulated and injected multiple times while attempting biliary cannulation. The bile duct is eventually cannulated only after performing a precut papillotomy using a needle-knife sphincterotome. In the recovery room, the patient appears uncomfortable and reports 10/10 epigastric pain radiating to the back. Abdominal X-ray does not reveal any free air or retroperitoneal air. WBC is 12.1K and lipase is 4000 U/L. Serum chemistries are normal. She is admitted to the hospital, and treated with IV fluids and analgesics. Her symptoms improve within 24 hours and she is discharged home on a low-fat diet.

▶ *What risk factors does this patient have for post-ERCP pancreatitis?*

▶ *What measures are recommended to reduce the risk of post-ERCP pancreatitis in this patient?*

▶ *How would you classify the severity of her pancreatitis?*

Vignette 12: Answer

The overall incidence of post-ERCP pancreatitis is only 2% to 4%. However, pancreatitis can occur in up to 40% of patients who have one of many predisposing risk factors; it's important to be very familiar with this list. Some of the factors are patient related, whereas others are procedure related. The most important patient related risk factors for post-ERCP pancreatitis are young age, female gender, suspected sphincter of Oddi dysfunction, and history of acute pancreatitis. Well-established procedure-related risk factors are ampullectomy and repeated pancreatic cannulation and injection. Patients undergoing sphincter of Oddi manometry also tend to have a high incidence of post-ERCP pancreatitis, but this is probably because they have several other risk factors and may not be entirely due to the manometry procedure itself. Similarly, post-ERCP pancreatitis after precut papillotomy in experienced hands is probably due to repeated cannulation attempts rather than the needle knife incision.

This young woman has a troubling "perfect storm" of converging risk factors which, when combined, place her at very high risk for post-ERCP pancreatitis. In addition to her predisposing demographics, she has suspected sphincter of Oddi dysfunction, experienced multiple attempts at cannulation, and underwent repeated pancreatic cannulations and injections.

Several measures can be employed to reduce the risk of post-ERCP pancreatitis. The traditional method of performing ERCP is to inject the duct with contrast prior to advancing the guidewire. Guidewire cannulation under fluoroscopy prior to contrast injection is associated with a reduced risk of pancreatitis compared to the traditional method, and is the preferred method of cannulation. If a pancreatogram is necessary, avoid overinjecting the pancreatic duct with contrast (visible on a pancreatogram as "acinarization," or filling of the pancreatic duct side branches—you don't want to see that if you can help it). This is because pressure from injection of contrast into the pancreatic duct can disrupt tight junctions between cells and lead to backflow of intraductal contents into the interstitial space and subsequent pancreatic injury. Spasm and stenosis of the major papilla following ERCP can obstruct flow of pancreatic duct contents leading to an increase in intraductal pressure and leakage into the interstitial space.

A pancreatic stent allows for drainage of pancreatic duct contents, and reduces the absolute risk of pancreatitis by about 10%. A temporary prophylactic pancreatic stent is therefore recommended in all high-risk patients undergoing ERCP. Randomized trials have also demonstrated a 10% absolute risk reduction with rectally administered nonsteroidal anti-inflammatory drugs (NSAIDs), particularly indomethacin or diclofenac.

This particular patient developed pancreatitis despite our placement of a prophylactic pancreatic stent and administration of rectal indomethacin at the end of the procedure. The most important preventive measure to reduce risk of post-ERCP pancreatitis is to avoid doing the ERCP to begin with (unless there is a strong indication for the procedure). That being said, pancreatic stents and rectal NSAIDs reduce the severity of pancreatitis as well.

Indeed, this patient was discharged home within 24 hours. She had no organ failure or local or systemic complications fitting the diagnosis of mild acute pancreatitis. Patients who develop transient organ failure that resolves within 24 to 48 hours or local or systemic complications (such as peripancreatic fluid collections) are classified as having moderately severe acute pancreatitis. Acute pancreatitis is classified as severe when there is persistent single or multiple organ failure lasting > 48 hours.

Since we're talking about acute pancreatitis, it's also worth knowing that Lactated Ringer's solution is the preferred crystalloid for intravenous hydration in acute pancreatitis. The rationale is that a lower pH level found in normal saline activates trypsinogen and makes acinar cells more susceptible to injury. Lactated Ringer's is more pH balanced and has a lower likelihood of hyperchloremic metabolic acidosis than normal saline solution. The exception is hypercalcemia-induced pancreatitis, where normal saline is preferred since Lactated Ringer's solution contains more calcium than normal saline solution. That's a nice point to remember for Board review.

Why Might This Be Tested? Pancreatitis is the most common severe complication of ERCP, and is the most common cause of ERCP related litigation. Recognizing which patients are at a higher risk for this complication is relevant for all gastroenterologists, even those who do not perform ERCP. In fact, go ahead and memorize the list of post-ERCP pancreatitis risk factors in Table 12-1, below. When you're done with that, go back and memorize it again. That's how important it is.

Clinical Threshold Alert: Amylase level should be at least 3 times the upper limit of normal to meet laboratory criteria for post-ERCP pancreatitis.

Table 12-1.
RISK FACTORS FOR DEVELOPING POST-ERCP PANCREATITIS
Post-ERCP Pancreatitis Risk Factors
• Suspected SOD (normal bili) • Female • Young (<50 years old) • Difficult cannulation • PD injection(s)—acinarization • Pancreatic sphincterotomy or PD therapy • Precut sphincterotomy, ampullectomy, balloon sphincteroplasty • Inexperienced endoscopist • History of acute pancreatitis

Here's the Point! 1

Know Table 12-1

Here's the Point! 2

Measures to reduce risk of post-ERCP pancreatitis are to avoid unnecessary ERCP in the first place, use guidewire cannulation, place a prophylactic pancreatic stent, and use rectal NSAIDs.

Here's the Point! 3

Lactated Ringer's solution is the preferred crystalloid for intravenous hydration in acute pancreatitis, except in hypercalcemia-induced pancreatitis.

Vignettes 13-20: ERCP Extravaganza

There's a good chance that your exam could feature one or more ERCP or MRCP images. If you become familiar with all the classics, then it will be easy to identify them quickly, answer the question correctly, and move on to harder stuff (like, how to diagnose ciguatera poisoning, or whatever craziness they throw at you next).

In this group of vignettes, called "ERCP Extravaganza," we've compiled 8 of the classics. We first show it to you in a simple, stylized, diagrammatic fashion to see if you can identify the abnormality. Then we show you an actual cholangiopancreatogram. We think it's more effective if you first learn the pared-down, simple diagram, and only then apply it to a real-life image. To kick things off, start by studying this simple diagram below:

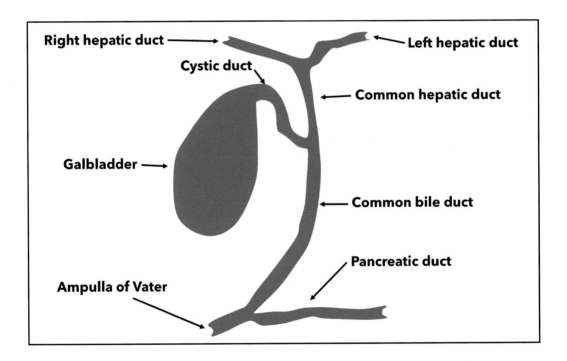

This much should be clear to you without further explanation (if not, then you're in trouble). There's the left and right hepatic ducts that converge to form the common hepatic duct. The common hepatic meets with the cystic duct to form the common bile duct (CBD). The CBD meets with the pancreatic duct (PD) to form a common channel that ends in the ampulla of Vater. Now, with that in mind, look at each of the following variants, and name the abnormality. Once you've given it your best shot, turn the page to see the answers.

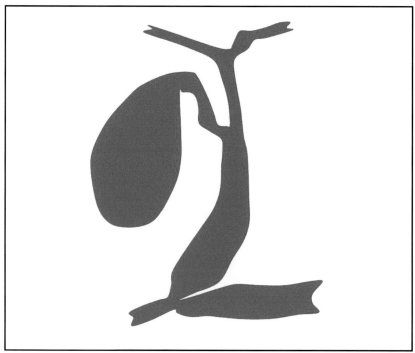

Vignette 13.

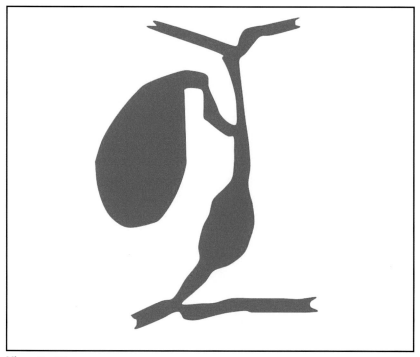

Vignette 14.

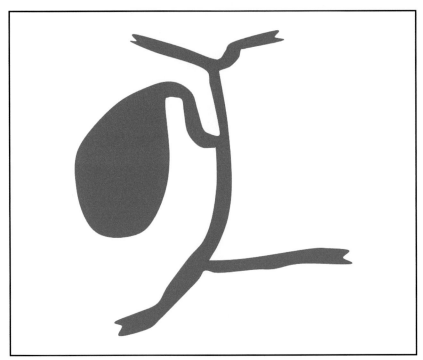

Vignette 15.

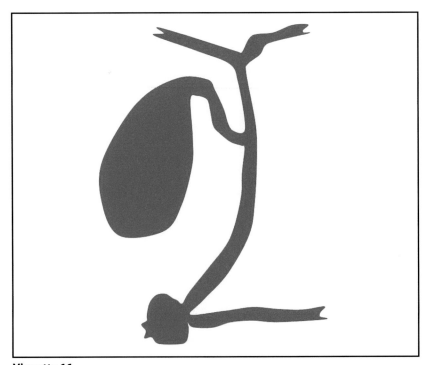

Vignette 16.

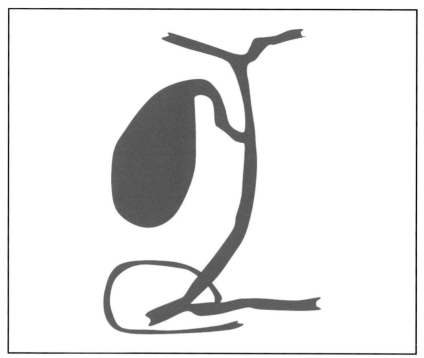

Vignette 17.

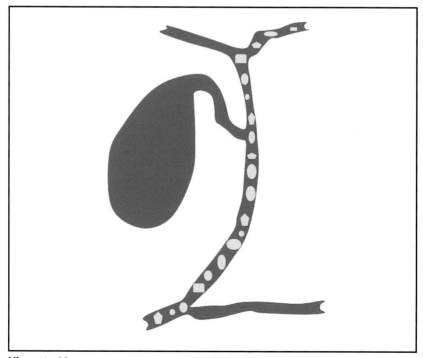

Vignette 18.

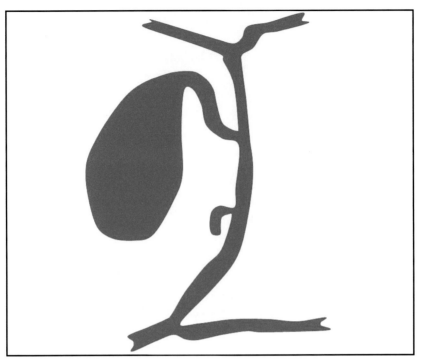

Vignette 19.

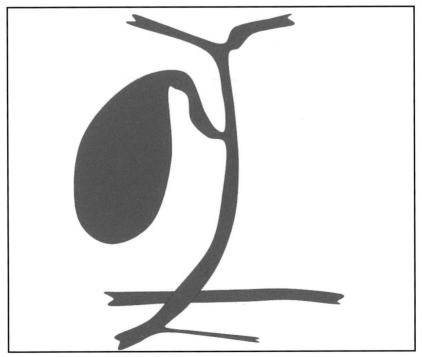

Vignette 20.

Vignettes 13-20: Answers

Okay, how did you do? Most of these are probably pretty easy, a few may have thrown you for a loop (literally, in the case of Vignette 17). Here are the answers, with corresponding real cholangiopancreatograms.

13. This is meant to show 2 dilated ducts—the CBD and PD. As we already covered in Vignette 8, this is the "double duct sign" and suggests there is a tumor simultaneously blocking both ducts. Figure 13-1 shows a corresponding MRCP image.

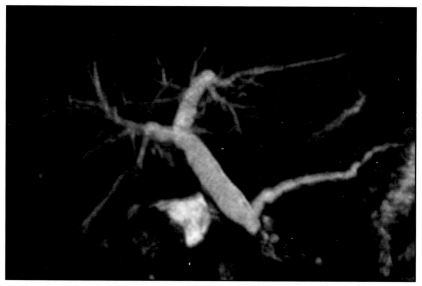

Figure 13-1. "Double duct sign" on MRCP.

14.   This is a type I choledochal cyst. Type I cysts are diffuse enlargements of the CBD and appear like a fusiform dilation along the CBD. There is a classic clinical triad associated with this and other choledochal cysts, marked by a palpable abdominal mass, jaundice, and abdominal pain. All choledochal cysts have malignant potential, and up to 30% of adult patients with bile duct cysts ultimately develop cholangiocarcinoma. The risk is higher with type I and II cysts (more later in the book), and lowest with type III cysts (also called choledochoceles—again, stay tuned). Refer to the first *Acing* book for a memory aid to distinguish amongst type I, II, and III cysts. Because the risk with type I and II cysts is substantial, it is generally recommended to surgically resect these particular cysts. Figure 14-1 shows a corresponding MRCP image.

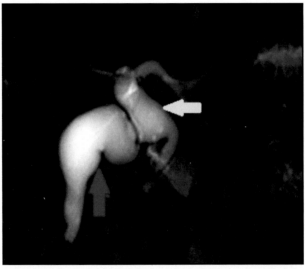

Figure 14-1. MRCP image of type I choledochal cyst with characteristic fusiform dilation of the extrahepatic bile duct (yellow arrow) with adjacent gallbladder (red arrow). (Reprinted with permission from Courtney Moreno, MD, Emory University.)

15. This is an anomalous panc-bil junction, or APBJ. Normally, the PD meets the CBD just before forming a short common channel ending with the ampulla of Vater. In this case, the PD inserts high up along the CBD, leaving a long, common channel where pancreatic juice can mix prematurely with bile. This is demonstrated in the ERCP shown below in Figure 15-1. It is important to know that this type of APBJ without concomitant choledochocele increases the risk for gallbladder cancer. So much so, that a prophylactic cholecystectomy is recommended in these patients. Often, choledochal cysts are associated with an APBJ, typically 2 cm or more from the sphincter of Oddi. The issue here is that the caustic pancreatic juices bathe the CBD and can reflux up into the proximal CBD. This can increase the risk of cholangiocarcinoma, which is why type I and type II cysts need to be managed aggressively with surgery.

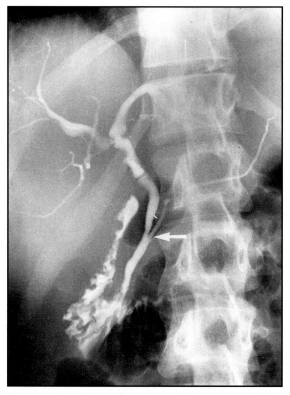

Figure 15-1. Anomalous panc-bil junction (APBJ). (Reprinted with permission from Anthony J. DiMarino Jr, MD and Stanley B. Benjamin, MD.)

16.   This is a type III choledochal cyst (aka "choledochocele"). Type III cysts are congenital dilations of the intraduodenal portion of the CBD. They appear as a bulging dilation at the end of the bile duct as it enters the duodenum. Choledochoceles have a lower malignant potential than type I and type II cysts with a malignant transformation risk of between 1% and 10%, depending on the series. Most authorities recommend endoscopic sphincterotomy as first-line therapy for symptomatic choledochoceles, reserving surgery for patients failing sphincterotomy or for those with recurrent complications like pancreatitis. Figure 16-1 shows a corresponding cholangiogram.

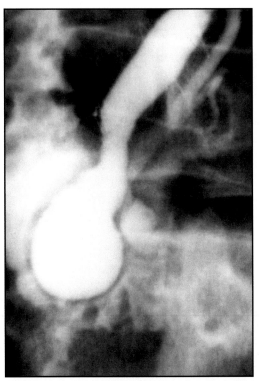

Figure 16-1. Type III choledochal cyst (also called a "choledochocele"). (Reprinted with permission from Mesleh M, Deziel DJ. Bile duct cysts. *Surg Clin North Am.* 2008;88:1369-1384.)

17. This is an annular pancreas. You can see that with the looping duct that runs around the duodenum and comes back again—a result of the ventral bud of the pancreas failing to migrate posteriorly during development. There is a classic radiographic sign that goes along with annular pancreas. Know what it is? Stay tuned, we'll cover annular pancreas in more detail later in the book. In the meantime, Figure 17-1 shows a characteristic ERCP image of annular pancreas, where the arrows point to a pancreatic duct ring.

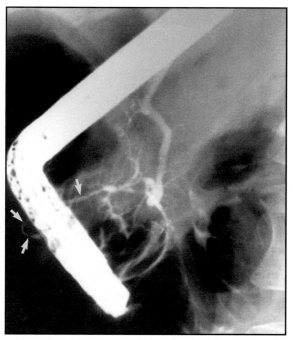

Figure 17-1. Annular pancreas. (Reprinted with permission from Anthony J. DiMarino Jr, MD and Stanley B. Benjamin, MD.)

18.   This is recurrent pyogenic cholangitis (previously termed "Oriental" cholangiohepatitis—
      a fortunately outdated name) with innumerable pigment stones piled up in the CBD and
      hepatic ductal systems. This condition, tends to occur almost exclusively in Asians. It has
      been linked to potential infectious etiologies, but the cause is still uncertain. The tip-off
      here is stones throughout the biliary system, including the hepatic ducts, with involvement
      of the left ductal system in particular (left side tends to be more commonly involved, pos-
      sibly due to tighter angulation vs the right ductal takeoff). You'll notice that the gallbladder
      has no stones, which is another key tipoff. Refer to the first *Acing* book for a more detailed
      discussion about recurrent pyogenic cholangitis, including its management. Figure 18-1
      shows a classic cholangiogram of this rare disorder.

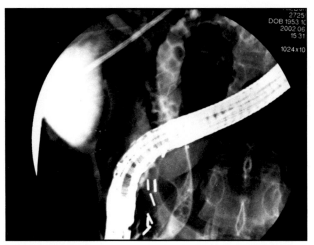

Figure 18-1. Recurrent pyogenic cholangitis with innumerable pigment biliary stones. (Reprinted with permission from
Francisco Durazo, MD, Ronald Reagan UCLA Medical Center.)

19. This is a type II choledochal cyst. Whereas type I cysts appear as a fusiform dilation of the CBD, type II cysts are small diverticula that stick off the side of the CBD. Take another look at it—you should be able to identify this one quite easily. See the original *Acing* book for more about these cysts if needed.

20. This is pancreas divisum, the most common congenial pancreatic anomaly. The pancreatogram reflects failure of the dorsal and ventral pancreatic ducts to fuse, so there is a small ventral duct draining through the major papilla, and a larger dorsal duct draining through the minor papilla. On imaging, the "crossing duct" sign is seen where the main pancreatic duct crosses the common bile duct to empty via the minor papilla. We cover pancreas divisum in more detail later in the book, including a cholangiopancreatogram, so we won't show the image or discuss management until later. Stay tuned.

Vignette 21: To ERCP... or not to ERCP?

A 38-year-old woman presents with acute onset of epigastric pain radiating to the back, along with nausea, and vomiting. She reports that over the last several months she has experienced episodes of right upper quadrant pain with meals that last less than 30 minutes. She does not consume any alcohol. On physical exam, she appears uncomfortable. Her epigastrium is diffusely tender to palpation. Vital signs are temperature 100.9°F, heart rate 114 beats/minute, and blood pressure 106/62 mm Hg. Laboratory studies are significant for WBC count of 12.9K, normal serum creatinine, normal serum calcium, normal triglycerides, serum lipase 4500 U/L, total bilirubin 3.2 mg/dL, alkaline phosphatase 306 U/L, AST 251 U/L, and ALT 286 U/L. Ultrasound reveals several gallstones, a 5-mm common bile duct, and no gallbladder wall thickening or pericholecystic fluid. Intravenous analgesia and hydration with Lactated Ringer's solution at 250 ml/hr is initiated. Twenty-four hours later, her vital signs are temperature 98.4°F, blood pressure 120/80 mm Hg, and heart rate 85 beats/minute. Repeat liver tests show total bilirubin 1.1 mg/dL, alkaline phosphatase 87 U/L, AST 32 U/L, ALT 31 U/L, and WBC 10.1K. You are consulted to perform an ERCP.

▶ **What is the next step in management?**

Vignette 21: Answer

This patient with gallstone pancreatitis initially presented with a high clinical suspicion for acute gallstone pancreatitis complicated by biliary obstruction and cholangitis (see predictors for CBD stones in Table 21-1). However, it is important to remember that acute pancreatitis can also cause fever, hypotension, and tachycardia (ie SIRS). With intravenous hydration, her vital signs have improved and liver tests have returned to the normal range. The patient likely had a common bile duct stone that passed spontaneously. An ERCP is not recommended in this setting (Table 21-2). The patient can safely undergo cholecystectomy once symptoms improve. In patients with mild acute gallstone pancreatitis, cholecystectomy should not be delayed by more than 1 to 2 weeks because failure to perform cholecystectomy carries a high risk for recurrent acute pancreatitis. Urgent ERCP within 24 hours would only have been indicated if the she had persistent signs of biliary obstruction and cholangitis. If her vital signs improved but liver tests remain significantly elevated, then an ERCP is warranted, but does not necessarily have to be performed urgently. By the way, what if this patient were, say, 28 weeks pregnant? Would you hold off on doing a cholecystectomy until after the delivery? We cover this scenario in the first *Acing* book and again later in this book, but in short, you need to operate then, too.

Why Might This Be Tested? Gastroenterologists are routinely consulted to perform an ERCP on patients with gallstone pancreatitis. You need to know when to "Just Say No."

Clinical Threshold Alert: Normal bile duct diameter in patients who have not undergone cholecystectomy is < 6 mm; normal bile duct diameter in elderly subjects is 1 mm per decade of life.

Table 21-1.	
PREDICTORS OF COMMON BILE DUCT STONES	
Very strong	• Common bile duct stone on ultrasound • Ascending cholangitis • Bilirubin > 4 mg/dL
Strong	• Dilated common bile duct on ultrasound (> 6 mm in patients with an intact gallbladder) • Bilirubin 1.8 to 4 mg/dL
Moderate	• Abnormal liver test other than bilirubin • Age > 55 years • Gallstone pancreatitis
Likelihood of CBD stones	• **High** = At least 1 very strong predictor, or at least 2 strong predictors • **Low** = no predictors • **Intermediate** = all other patients

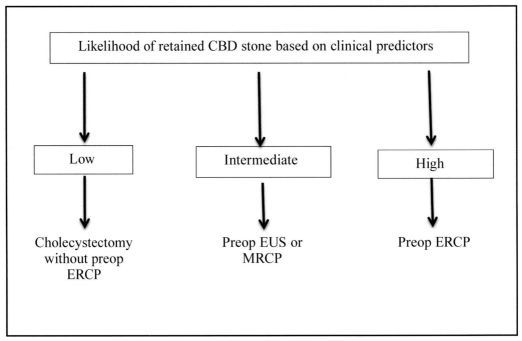

Table 21-2. Management algorithm for CBD stones based on clinical probability.

Here's the Point! 1

Gallstone pancreatitis + Liver tests return to normal = Can safely perform cholecystectomy without preoperative ERCP

Here's the Point! 2

The only indication for urgent ERCP in gallstone pancreatitis is acute cholangitis.

Vignette 22: Feeding Frenzy

A 47-year-old man with a history of heavy alcohol use presents to the emergency department with acute onset of severe gnawing epigastric pain radiating to the back, nausea, and vomiting. Vital signs are temperature 100.2°F, blood pressure 80/60 mm Hg, and heart rate 120 beats/minute. On exam, he appears uncomfortable with epigastric tenderness to palpation. Laboratory studies are significant for WBC count of 13K, creatinine of 2.7 mg/dL, and serum lipase 5390 U/L. Liver tests and triglycerides are normal. There are no gallstones, pericholecystic fluid, or gallbladder wall thickening on transabdominal ultrasound. Intravenous analgesia and hydration with boluses of Lactated Ringer's solution are initiated. He remains hypotensive despite 4 L of Lactated Ringer's, and is therefore admitted to the intensive care unit. You have told the ICU nurse that you are planning to feed the patient, but the nurse is in a frenzy about this and wants clarification before carrying out your orders.

▶ *When should you start feeding this patient?*

▶ *If so, what feeding route should you use?*

Vignette 22: Answer

You should initiate enteral nutrition via nasogastric tube right away in this patient with severe acute pancreatitis. You may have learned the dictum to "let the pancreas rest" when it's inflamed and avoid any stimulation of the exocrine pancreas. Many of us learned to approach the pancreas like a big, gnarly, sleeping dog we didn't want to poke with a stick. Turns out that was pretty much wrong. In fact, in some cases that advice was dead wrong. Bowel rest can lead to intestinal atrophy, which increases the risk of infectious complications due to bacterial translocation across the gut— that's the last thing a patient with acute pancreatitis needs during their most vulnerable state. In contrast, early initiation of enteral feeding within 24 hours reduces infectious complications and decreases mortality in patients with severe acute pancreatitis. Parenteral nutrition is not recommended because it does not maintain the gut barrier in a similar fashion to enteral nutrition, and predisposes to significant risks, including catheter sepsis.

Enteral nutrition was traditionally provided via nasojejunal tube (NJT) to avoid the gastric phase of stimulation and reduce the risk of pulmonary aspiration. The idea was to tip-toe the food past the sleeping dog (ie the pancreas) and deliver it downstream via NJT. However, NJTs do not eliminate the risk of aspiration. Moreover, nasogastric tubes (NGTs) provide comparable efficacy and safety as NJTs, and are cheaper and less cumbersome to place than a NJT. So, the NGT feeding route is fine.

Clinical trials assessing the role of nutrition in acute pancreatitis have often used a peptide based semielemental formula that is high in protein and low in fat. In practice, a standard formula is typically used first. Because of this variation in clinical practice, you probably won't be asked what type of enteral feed to initiate. It is more important to feed with what you've got.

In mild acute pancreatitis, you should start an oral diet as soon as it can be tolerated (usually within 24 to 48 hours). Just keep an eye out for ileus, which can accompany pancreatitis, although not typical for mild disease. Initiating feeding with a low-fat diet is probably as safe as a clear liquid diet. Switching to enteral feeding is recommended in mild acute pancreatitis if the patient cannot tolerate an oral diet by 7 days.

Why Might This Be Tested? Contrary to prior belief, early initiation of enteral feeding is safe in severe acute pancreatitis and reduces mortality. You should be aware of this important shift in the treatment paradigm for severe acute pancreatitis. By the way, we don't want you actually poking dogs with sticks; that was an analogy. So, don't poke dogs with sticks, and let sleeping dogs lie. But do feed patients with acute pancreatitis. Not sure how we got to talking about dogs. But studying for Boards is painfully boring, so at least we're having fun now talking about dogs. Maybe. Anyway...

Here's the Point!

Initiate enteral feeding via NGT within 24 hours in severe acute pancreatitis. NJT is not required.

Vignette 23: Is My Sphincter Tight?

A 40-year-old woman is seen in consultation for evaluation of recurrent acute pancreatitis. She had a cholecystectomy for biliary dyskinesia two years ago, and has not had biliary symptoms since that time. She has no other medical problems. In between episodes of acute pancreatitis, she remains asymptomatic. She does not take any medications or over the counter drugs. She does not smoke cigarettes, drink alcohol, or use any illicit drugs. She does not have a family history of autoimmune conditions, pancreatitis, or pancreatic cancer. Her laboratory evaluation for etiologies of acute pancreatitis has been unrevealing, including normal calcium, normal triglycerides, normal ANA and IgG4, and negative testing for hereditary pancreatitis. MRI does not reveal any pancreatic mass, and the bile duct and pancreatic ducts are normal. An endoscopic ultrasound is performed and does not reveal an occult pancreatic mass, periampullary diverticulum, ampullary mass, or biliary sludge. The patient undergoes ERCP with sphincter of Oddi manometry to further evaluate her symptoms. The peak pressures are noted to be 60 to 80 mm Hg, with nadir pressure sustained at 10 to 30 mm Hg in all leads.

▶ *How do you interpret the sphincter of Oddi manometry findings?*

▶ *What is the next step in management based on the manometry findings?*

Vignette 23: Answer

Before delving into the interpretation of the manometry findings, it's worth getting into a little bit of detail about the sphincter of Oddi (SO). Controversy has mired this poor little muscle since its original description over 100 years ago. Most recently, Rome IV guidelines completely redefined SO disorders (SOD), and management recommendations have also changed, particularly regarding the previously termed type 3 SOD.

The SO is comprised of tonically active smooth muscle located at the end of the bile duct and pancreatic duct. During feeding, cholecystokinin as well as other hormones and neurally-mediated reflexes stimulate gallbladder contraction and pancreatic secretion as well as relaxation of the SO. This coordinated activity allows bile and pancreatic secretions to enter the duodenal lumen to facilitate digestion and absorption. Disordered relaxation of the pancreatic SO could therefore predispose to recurrent acute pancreatitis.

Patients with recurrent episodes of otherwise unexplained pancreatitis and main pancreatic duct dilation likely have pancreatic sphincter of Oddi stenosis (previously termed type 1 pancreatic SOD). These patients have a high enough likelihood of benefitting from pancreatic sphincterotomy that further testing with sphincter of Oddi manometry is not warranted. Our patient with unexplained recurrent acute pancreatitis without pancreatic duct dilation could have functional pancreatic SOD, previously termed type 2 SOD. In this case, Rome IV guidelines do endorse SO manometry to assess whether a pancreatic sphincterotomy can provide symptomatic relief. Manometry is considered abnormal if the nadir pressure is sustainably elevated to > 40 mm Hg in both leads across multiple stations. In this case, peak pressures are elevated to > 40 mm Hg, but the nadir pressures are < 40 mm Hg. This is a normal pancreatic sphincter of Oddi manometry tracing. A pancreatic sphincterotomy is unlikely to benefit this patient. So, 40 is the magic number and you need to pay attention to the nadir measurement. Also, don't forget about the high risk of post-ERCP pancreatitis in this young female with a history of recurrent acute pancreatitis and suspected SOD (check out Vignette 12 again). To reduce her risk of post-ERCP pancreatitis, she should be considered for a temporary prophylactic pancreatic stent and rectal NSAIDs.

Why Might This Be Tested? Suspected SOD is a common reason patients are referred to panc-bil clinics in tertiary care centers. Whether you are the referring GI or panc-bil expert, you should recognize when sphincterotomy without manometry is sufficient (sphincter of Oddi stenosis) and when an ERCP is more likely to harm your patients than help them (type 3 SOD). Board examiners don't want you performing unnecessary ERCPs (nor do your lawyers).

Clinical Threshold Alert 1: Normal pancreatic duct diameter is up to 3 mm in the head, 2 mm in the body, and 1 mm in the tail of the pancreas. You can think of it as the "3, 2, 1 Rule" (but not the "3, 2, 1 Rule" of the Bethesda Criteria; that's in another *Acing* book!).

Clinical Threshold Alert 2: Sphincter of Oddi manometry is considered abnormal when the nadir pressure is sustainably elevated to > 40 mm Hg in both leads across multiple stations.

Here's the Point!

Unexplained recurrent acute pancreatitis + Dilated pancreatic duct = Pancreatic sphincter of Oddi stenosis (previously termed type 1 SOD) → Perform pancreatic sphincterotomy without manometry

Vignette 24: Divided We Fall

You are excited to see a 31-year-old woman in the clinic for chief complaint of chronic abdominal pain. For over a decade, she reports generalized, persistent discomfort that worsens with meals and improves after a bowel movement. She also reports constipation alternating with diarrhea. She has had a 5-lb weight gain over the last 12 months. Vital signs are temperature 98.3°F, blood pressure 118/75 mm Hg, pulse 75 beats/minute, and oxygen saturation 99% on room air. On physical examination, the patient is well appearing and in no acute distress. She has mild diffuse abdominal tenderness to palpation without rebound or guarding. She has brought records from prior evaluations, which include a normal complete blood count, normal serum chemistry, normal amylase and lipase, normal liver tests, and normal thyroid tests. As part of the evaluation, MRCP was obtained (Figure 24-1).

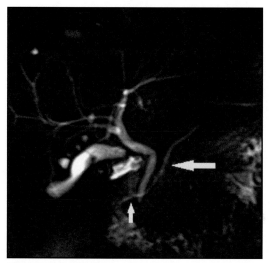

Figure 24-1. MRCP image.

▶ *What anomaly is present on the patient's MRI?*

▶ *Is an ERCP warranted?*

Vignette 24: Answer

The anomaly seen on MRCP is pancreas divisum, the most common congenital pancreatic anomaly with an approximate 7% prevalence in the general population. This anomaly results from failure of the dorsal and ventral pancreatic ducts to fuse. The classic pancreas divisum anatomy is a small ventral duct that drains through the major papilla, and a larger dorsal duct that drains through the minor papilla. Look at that image again. Did you see the "crossing duct sign" where the pancreatic duct (arrows in Figure 24-1) crosses the common bile duct to drain through the minor papilla? Since the minor papilla is smaller than the major papilla, the dorsal duct may not adequately drain, which can produce high intraductal pressure, dorsal ductal distension, and consequently pancreatic type pain and even pancreatitis. However, less than 5% of patients with pancreas divisum report pancreatic pain symptoms. Moreover, the incidence of pancreas divisum does not differ between patients with and without pancreatitis. You got that? We used to think that pancreas divisum was a big risk factor for pancreatitis; but, we now know that's not the reality.

Patients with pancreas divisum who have recurrent acute pancreatitis and pancreatic-type pain may benefit from ERCP with cannulation of the minor papilla and minor papillotomy. You don't need to learn the technical nuances of achieving minor papilla cannulation for Board review. However, you should know that it's hard to find the minor papilla. To facilitate identification of a diminutive minor papilla, you can spray methylene blue (surrounding mucosa will stain blue, while the minor papilla does not stain) or administer intravenous secretin. Surgical sphincteroplasty is an option if minor papilla cannulation is unsuccessful or papillotomy is incomplete. This patient's pain is more consistent with irritable bowel syndrome than related to pancreatic duct outflow obstruction. For her, pancreas divisum is probably a coincidental finding of no clinical consequence. Minor papillotomy is very unlikely to provide any clinical benefit, so the risk of performing an ERCP in this case is not justified. You better call a good lawyer if you're even thinking about an ERCP. You don't want to "divide" the sphincter in this case of divisum, or eventually "divided we'll fall" (…into court with your patient). ☹

Why Might This Be Tested? Pancreas divisum is the most common congenital anomaly of the pancreas and is therefore not an uncommon finding. Like many other incidental findings, pancreas divisum usually remains asymptomatic in the vast majority. Not every patient with pancreas divisum benefits from an ERCP, so this condition requires radiology interpretation as well as management of radiology findings. It's a good way to see if you're trigger-happy with ERCP. Remember, it's hard to cause serious problems with a colonoscopy or endoscopy, but ERCP can have serious consequences, so use it wisely.

Here's the Point! 1

Pancreas divisum + Recurrent acute pancreatitis → Perform ERCP and minor papillotomy

Here's the Point! 2

ERCP is not indicated for incidentally detected pancreas divisum.

Vignette 25: A Fluid Situation

A 45-year-old man presents to the emergency department with acute onset of severe gnawing epigastric pain radiating to the back. He has a longstanding history of heavy alcohol use with no other medical problems. Vital signs on admission are temperature 100.5°F, blood pressure 105/68 mm Hg, and heart rate 99 beats/minute. On exam, he has significant tenderness to palpation in the epigastrium. Serum lipase is 3900 U/L and WBC count is 10.8K. Serum liver tests, chemistry, calcium, and triglyceride levels are normal. There are no stones or sludge on gallbladder ultrasound. He is admitted to the hospital and hydrated with Lactated Ringer's solution. After 48 hours, vital signs are normal and he is tolerating a low-fat diet. However, he continues to experience persistent abdominal pain so a CT scan is obtained (Figure 25-1). On review of his records, he had presented to the emergency department 3 months ago with abdominal discomfort, and a CT scan obtained at that time was normal.

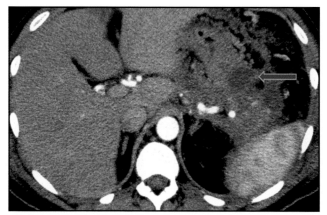

Figure 25-1. CT scan. (Reprinted with permission from Tenner S, Brown A, Gress FG. *Curbside Consultation of the Pancreas: 49 Clinical Questions.* Thorofare, NJ: SLACK Incorporated; 2010.)

▶ *What is this finding called?*

▶ *How should you manage this?*

Vignette 25: Answer

This patient has acute pancreatitis with an acute peripancreatic fluid collection (APFC), which is seen on this CT scan (arrow in Figure 25-1). APFCs usually develop in the early phase of pancreatitis and are disorganized without a well-defined wall. For this otherwise stable patient with an APFC, no specific intervention is recommended at this time, since most APFCs resolve spontaneously within 7 to 10 days.

In 4 to 6 weeks however, this patient should undergo repeat cross-sectional imaging since 15% of APFCs do persist. That is, over the course of 4 to 6 weeks, persistent APFCs organize into a fluid collection with a well-defined wall (Figure 25-2)—ie a pseudocyst. The "pseudo" in pseudocyst distinguishes the lesion from real cysts which are lined by epithelial tissue. In contrast, a pseudocyst is not lined by epithelium, but instead is lined by compacted pancreatic parenchyma and granulation tissue squished together. If the patient develops a pseudocyst but is otherwise asymptomatic, then you can counsel the patient that an intervention is not necessary because 40% of pseudocysts resolve without any specific intervention. Observation and repeat imaging such as a CT scan in 3 to 6 months is sufficient for an asymptomatic patient with a pseudocyst. Bear in mind, this is different from previous guidelines that called for drainage of large (ie >6 cm) cysts or those persisting for a while (ie >6 weeks) after acute pancreatitis. No matter the size or durability, if a patient is doing fine and there are no obvious complications, then you shouldn't rush into draining the lesion.

Some patients with a pseudocyst may develop symptoms of abdominal pain, or complications such as infection, pseudoaneurysm, or biliary obstruction from cyst expansion. For small complicated pseudocysts <6 cm that communicate with the main pancreatic duct, placement of a pancreatic duct stent (transpapillary drainage) may be sufficient. For larger complicated pseudocysts, options are endoscopic, surgical, or percutaneous drainage. The decision of a particular technique or modality is often guided by local expertise. Endoscopic drainage is the least invasive, but requires that the cyst abuts the gastric or duodenal wall, and is contraindicated in patients with a pseudoaneurysm. Percutaneous drainage can be helpful for some but may lead to pancreaticocutaneous fistula formation. Surgery is obviously the most invasive method of drainage.

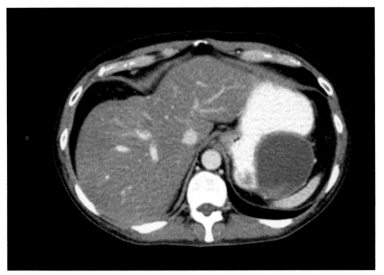

Figure 25-2. Pancreatic pseudocyst.

Why Might This Be Tested? APFCs are common, and occur in one-half to two-thirds of acute pancreatitis. Gastroenterologists are consulted to help guide management when APFCs occur. Also, the old surgical dictum that all pseudocysts that persist >6 weeks or are >6 cm in diameter require surgery is no longer considered valid. Remember that patience for patients is a virtue.

Here's the Point! 1

Acute pancreatitis + Unorganized fluid collections around pancreas in first few days = Acute peripancreatic fluid collection

Here's the Point! 2

Prior history of pancreatitis + Walled off fluid collection = Pseudocyst

Vignette 26: WhOPpiN' Pain

A 52-year-old man is admitted with severe epigastric pain radiating to the back. He does not drink any alcohol or smoke cigarrettes. Vital signs are temperature 100.8°F, blood pressure 98/78 mm Hg, pulse 110 beats/minute, and oxygen saturation 95% on room air. WBC count is 12.1K and serum lipase is 5120 U/L. Serum chemistry, liver tests, calcium, and triglyceride levels are normal. Gallbladder ultrasound demonstrates several large gallstones as well as sludge but no bile duct dilation. He is admitted to the hospital and intravenous analgesia and intravenous fluids are initiated. Despite several days of bowel rest and IV Lactated Ringer's solution, he continues to complain of "whopping" abdominal pain and is unable to tolerate an oral diet. An MRI of the abdomen is obtained and demonstrates nonenhancement of at least 50% of the pancreatic tissue, and an unorganized fluid collection with solid material. Vital signs are temperature 97.1°F, blood pressure 120/80 mm Hg, and heart rate 95 beats/minute. WBC count is 8.5K and serum lipase is 25 U/L.

▶ *What's the diagnosis?*

▶ *What should you do next?*

Vignette 26: Answer

The patient has acute necrotizing pancreatitis complicated by a necrotic fluid collection. Pancreatic necrosis is visible on CT or MRI contrast imaging as areas of nonenhancement of the pancreatic gland. Necrosis within a peripancreatic fluid collection appears as solid material within the fluid collection. To meet the definition of necrotizing pancreatitis, at least 30% or 3 cm of the pancreatic parenchyma should fail to enhance (ie nonviable tissue). Necrosis with no signs of infection is termed sterile necrosis and is generally less concerning. Although sterile necrosis can still become infected, prophylactic antibiotics are not recommended (this is a change from historical practice of treating all necrotic tissue with empirical antibiotics). This patient with sterile necrosis should undergo repeat cross-sectional contrast imaging in 6 weeks and does not need antibiotics now.

In patients who develop signs of infected necrosis, reasonable options include empiric antibiotics vs EUS or CT guided FNA for gram stain and culture—both options are acceptable. If you select an empiric antibiotic strategy, use an intravenous antibiotic that penetrates pancreatic necrosis (such as carbapenems, quinolones, metronidazole, and high dose cephalosporins). As long as the patient is clinically stable, try to avoid debridement of infected or symptomatic necrosis until the necrotic fluid collection becomes organized over the next 6 weeks into a walled off pancreatic necrosis (WOPN).

Once a WOPN forms as a more consolidated, walled off mass (previously termed a "phlegmon"), it becomes easier to debride. You should also know that minimally invasive methods of debridement (endoscopic or percutaneous) are preferred to surgical debridement because surgery carries a higher risk of complications and death. In contrast, if the necrotic tissue is not walled off and/or the patient is clinically unstable, then a surgical approach is generally preferred. As an aside, know that severe or necrotizing pancreatitis is a reasonable indication to delay cholecystectomy in gallstone pancreatitis; that's a nice little pearl.

Okay, let's review. Management of pancreatic necrosis is very algorithmic and Figure 26-1 provides a step-by-step algorithm of how to approach pancreatic necrosis for both Board review and real life. Start by figuring out if the patient is clinically stable. If you have a patient with pancreatic necrosis who is hypotensive and looking really sick, then call a surgeon. But if the patient is clinically stable, you've got some time. Figure out if the necrosis appears infected or not, using the approaches described above. If it's sterile necrosis, then don't use antibiotics and carefully monitor the patient for signs of clinical decompensation or infection (or both). If the necrosis appears infected but the patient is clinicaly stable, then determine if it's liquefied or walled off (ie WOPN). If it's liquefied, then you need to start antibiotics but it's premature to do a necrosectomy. If you've got a symptomatic WOPN, then do a necrosectomy but stay away from the surgeons if you can—preferentially do an endoscopic or percutaneous procedure.

Why Might This Be Tested? In the past, antibiotics were routinely recommended in patients with sterile necrosis and surgery was the primary method of debridement. There is strong evidence that patients with sterile necrosis do not require prophylactic antibiotics, and that minimally invasive debridement provides better outcomes than surgery. So, you gotta stay with the times! You want to make sure your practice is consistent with the current standard of care and you're not holding onto old dogma that is not evidence-based.

Clinical Threshold Alert: Necrotizing pancreatitis = Nonviable pancreatic parenchyma of at least 30% or 3 cm.

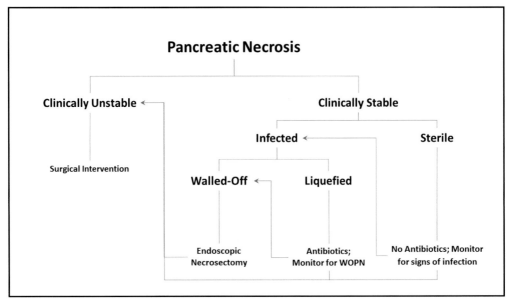

Figure 26-1. Algorithm for managing pancreatic necrosis.

Here's the Point!

Pancreatitis + Nonenhancement of > 30% of pancreatic parenchyma on contrast-enhanced cross-sectional imaging = Necrotizing pancreatitis

Vignette 27: A Growth Spurt

A 55-year-old man undergoes repeat CT scan with oral and IV contrast 3 months after an episode of acute pancreatitis complicated by an acute peripancreatic fluid collection. He is currently asymptomatic. This CT scan reveals a 4-cm x 3-cm walled off fluid collection without solid material. Four weeks pass by. He then presents with acute onset of severe epigastric pain radiating to the left flank, with nausea, and vomiting. On examination, he appears pale and uncomfortable, with epigastric and left upper quadrant abdominal tenderness. Vital signs are temperature 96.9°F, blood pressure 70/50 mm Hg, heart rate 120 beats/minute. Laboratory studies are significant for WBC count of 8.9K, hemoglobin 5.1 g/dL, platelets 181K, creatinine 2.1 mg/dL, and lipase 10 U/L. Liver tests are normal. Aggressive intravenous hydration is initiated and another CT scan is obtained. The cyst has now increased in size to 9 cm x 7 cm, and there is high density material within the cyst.

▶ *What's going on here?*

▶ *What are you going to do next?*

Vignette 27: Answer

The patient has a ruptured pseudoaneurysm—that's big time trouble! A pseudoaneurysm occurred here due to a pseudocyst eroding into the wall of a pancreatic or peripancreatic artery, leading to a communication between the artery and the pseudocyst. They are termed pseudoaneuryms because the vessel wall is lined by fibrous tissue rather than endothelial cells. Pseudoaneurysms occur in approximately 10% of walled off pancreatic fluid collections with the most commonly involved vessels being the splenic, hepatic, gastroduodenal, and pancreaticoduodenal arteries.

Occasionally, autodigestion of the pseudoaneurysm wall by pancreatic enzymes can lead to rupture. You should suspect this complication when a patient with a walled off pancreatic fluid collection presents with sudden drop in hemoglobin and rapid expansion of the fluid collection—ie a "growth spurt." Pseudoaneurysm rupture is a severe, life-threatening complication (just think about arterial spurting!) that requires emergent intervention. The 2 options for intervention are mesenteric angiography with selective embolization, and surgical ligation. Also, you should know that an untreated pseudoaneurym is an absolute contraindication to endoscopic pseudocyst drainage due to the high risk of severe and fatal hemorrhage. You don't want to be putting any sharp instruments through that! There is another acute presentation for pseudoaneurysm rupture. Stay tuned...

Why Might This Be Tested? Ruptured pseudoaneursym is an uncommon but life-threatening complication of pancreatitis. Prompt recognition and emergent intervention can make the difference between life and death for the patient.

Here's the Point!

Acute abdominal pain + Pallor + Sudden expansion of pseudocyst = Ruptured pseudoaneurysm

Vignette 28: A Sinistral Problem

A 54-year-old is admitted to the hospital with severe epigastric pain radiating to the back. He has a history of heavy alcohol use. Vital signs are temperature 100.2°F, blood pressure 100/80 mm Hg, heart rate 102 beats/minute, and oxygen saturation 98% on room air. WBC count is 11.4K, hemoglobin is 13 g/dL, platelet count 194K, serum lipase is 6000 U/L, serum chemistry and liver tests are normal. Serum calcium and triglycerides are normal. Right upper quadrant ultrasound does not reveal any stones or sludge. He is admitted to the hospital and treated with intravenous fluids and analgesics. His symptoms improve and he is discharged within 48 hours with minimal abdominal discomfort and is tolerating a low-fat diet. One week later, he presents to the emergency department with hematemesis. He has not had any alcohol since he was discharged. Vital signs are temperature 98.4°F, blood pressure 80/60 mm Hg, and pulse 120 beats/minute. Serum hemoglobin is 7 g/dL. He receives intravenous fluids, blood transfusion, and undergoes an upper endoscopy. Endoscopy reveals isolated gastric varices with red wale signs but without active bleeding. There is no portal hypertensive gastropathy or esophageal varices.

▶ *What is going on here?*

▶ *How should you treat with complication?*

Vignette 28: Answer

It may be tempting to conclude that the patient's varices are related to portal hypertension from alcoholic cirrhosis. However, he has no portal hypertensive gastropathy or esophageal varices and lack of thrombocytopenia argues against portal hypertension. So, this particular patient with pancreatitis and isolated gastric varices likely has splenic vein thrombosis. The splenic vein courses directly posterior to the body and tail of the pancreas. Due to its location, inflammation from pancreatitis can lead to perivenous inflammation and thrombosis. Splenic vein thrombosis results in extrahepatic, sinistral (left-sided) portal hypertension. As a result, blood flows retrograde through the short and posterior gastric veins and the gastroepiploic veins resulting in the formation of gastric varices. Pancreatitis is the most common cause of splenic vein thrombosis, and splenic vein thrombosis is the most common cause of isolated gastric varices. Other potential etiologies for splenic vein thrombosis include hypercoagulability, and splenic vein obstruction from pseudocysts and lymph nodes.

Interestingly, the risk of bleeding from isolated gastric varices due to splenic vein thrombosis is quite low. Observation without any specific intervention is reasonable in patients with asymptomatic gastric varices due to splenic vein thrombosis, particularly if the varices are seen on CT scan but not on endoscopy. When bleeding does occur, splenectomy is the treatment of choice. Splenectomy eliminates venous collateral outflow and thereby decompresses surrounding varices.

For more detailed review of this entity, including a thorough review of the underlying anatomy, refer to the hepatology book in the *Acing* series.

Why Might This Be Tested? This topic allows relationship and understanding of 2 major GI topics, pancreatitis and GI bleeding. Also, its important to recognize that the treatment of isolated gastric varices due to splenic vein thrombosis differs from cirrhosis-related variceal bleeding.

Here's the Point!

Pancreatitis + Isolated gastric varices = Splenic vein thrombosis

Vignettes 29-33: Name That Cyst!

Pancreatic cysts are identified in 1% of all cross-sectional abdominal imaging tests, and are a common reason for gastroenterology consultations. Differentiating the type of cystic neoplasm is clinically important because the malignant potential of these cysts ranges from negligible to very high. Pancreatic cystic neoplasms have characteristic epidemiologic, imaging, and fine needle aspirate findings, which makes them ideal fodder for Board review. There are also a bunch of Board "buzzwords" associated with pancreas cysts, so knowing them will help you that much more. For each vignette below, identify the most likely pancreatic cystic neoplasm, and the malignant potential of each neoplasm.

29. A middle-aged woman is incidentally found to have a 3-cm cyst in the head of the pancreas, which has a microcystic ("honeycomb") appearance.

30. A 23-year-old woman is incidentally found to have a 2-cm pancreatic head cyst.

31. A middle-aged man is incidentally noted to have several small cysts in the head and body of the pancreas. The main pancreatic duct is not dilated and the cysts do not communicate with the main pancreatic duct either. FNA of the largest 2.8-cm cyst yields 2 mL of thick viscous fluid. Carcinoembryonic antigen (CEA) is 1000 ng/mL and amylase is 1200 U/L.

32. A 60-year-old man with 2 episodes of idiopathic pancreatitis is found to have a 4-cm cyst in the head of the pancreas. The cyst communicates with the main pancreatic duct. During side-viewing examination with a duodenoscope, the major papilla appears patulous with mucin extruding from the papilla.

33. A 60-year-old woman is incidentally found to have a 3-cm cyst in the tail of the pancreas. The cyst does not communicate with the head of the pancreas. FNA reveals a CEA of 1800 ng/mL.

Vignettes 29-33: Answers

29.   The patient has a serous cystadenoma. Serous cystadenomas can occur anywhere in the pancreas, and typically occur in middle-aged women, although they can occur in men. The characteristic imaging appearance of a serous cystadenoma is a microcystic ("honeycomb") appearance, often with a central scar. FNA typically yields thin, serosanguinous fluid. Because this lesion does not contain mucin, the CEA level is typically low. Serous cystadenomas do not communicate with the pancreatic duct, so the amylase level is normal. Glycogen staining of the cyst fluid is often positive, and cytology may demonstrate cuboidal cells. This type of cyst grows slowly over time, but its malignant potential is negligible. Surveillance is unnecessary once a diagnosis of a serous cystadenoma is firmly established.

By the way, can you name 2 liver lesions with a central scar? See the hepatology book in the *Acing* series for a refresher if needed.

Here's the Point!

Pancreatic cyst + Microcystic ("honeycomb") appearance + Low CEA = Serous cystadenoma (negligible malignant potential)

30.   You probably noticed that this vignette did not provide any information except the patient's age and gender. This is because pancreatic cystic neoplasms typically occur in middle-aged patients between the fifth to seventh decade with one notable exception. Solid pseudopapillary neoplasms tend to occur in younger women (second to third decade). FNA typically yields bloody fluid and cytology may show branching finger-like projections (pseudopapillae). This lesion's malignant potential is in the moderate to even high range over the long time course as this often presents at a young age.

Here's the Point!

Young woman with pancreatic cyst = Probably a solid pseudopapillary neoplasm

31. This is a branch-duct intraductal papillary mucinous neoplasm (IPMN). Because these lesions arise from a branch of the pancreatic duct, the amylase level is high. And because they contain mucin, the CEA level will be high too. Unlike IPMNs that arise from the main pancreatic duct, the malignant potential of branch-duct IPMNs is low to moderate, so surveillance rather than resection is a reasonable strategy if the largest cyst is less than 3 cm, the main pancreatic duct is not dilated and none of the cysts contain a solid component ("mural nodule"). The frequency of surveillance is controversial and is therefore not as pertinent for Board review. What you should know is that branch-duct IPMNs look like a "cluster of grapes" on imaging due to the multiple dilated side branches. Refer to the original *Acing* book for a more detailed review of IPMNs and their management.

Here's the Point! 1

Cyst amylase level is elevated if the lesion communicates with the pancreatic duct (IPMNs and pseudocysts)

Here's the Point! 2

CEA level is elevated in cysts that contain mucin (IPMNs, mucinous cystic neoplasms)

32. This is a main-duct IPMN. A classic finding on side-viewing examination is a patulous major papilla with mucin extruding from the ampulla ("fish mouth deformity"), as shown in Figure 32-1. Like branch-duct IPMNs, these lesions occur equally frequently in males and females. Also similar to branch-duct IPMNs, the main-duct IPMNs typically have an elevated CEA and amylase level in the cyst aspirate, and cytology may yield columnar cells. However, unlike branch-duct IPMNs, the main-duct IPMNs carry a significantly higher malignant potential. Therefore, surgical resection should be offered to all surgically fit patients with a main-duct IPMN.

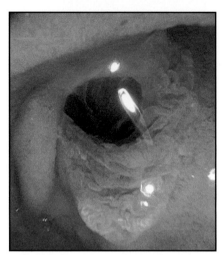

Figure 32-1. Fish mouth ampulla of main duct IPMN.

Here's the Point!

Pancreatic cyst + Communication with the main pancreatic duct + "Fish mouth" deformity = Main-duct IPMN (very high malignant potential)

33. This is probably a mucinous cystic neoplasm (MCN). Although an IPMN is also possible, they tend to occur more frequently in the head of the pancreas, whereas MCNs are more commonly located in the body and tail. In addition, unlike IPMNs, MCNs almost exclusively occur in females. However, in parallel to IMPNs, MCNs contain mucin so cyst fluid aspirate should yield an elevated CEA. In theory, the amylase level should be low since the cyst does not communicate with the pancreatic duct. However, the amylase level does not reliably differentiate IPMNs from MCNs. MCNs have a malignant potential that is higher than branch-duct IPMNs but lower than main-duct IPMNs. Surgical resection should be considered for acceptable surgical candidates.

Clinical Threshold Alert: CEA > 192 ng/mL in pancreatic cyst fluid accurately differentiates a mucinous from a nonmucinous neoplasm. The CEA level in pancreatic cyst fluid is not predictive of malignancy.

Here's the Point!

- **Gender: IPMNs occur equally frequently in males and females; mucinous cystic neoplasms almost exclusively occur in females.**
- **Location: IPMNs are more commonly located in the head; mucinous cystic neoplasms typically occur in the body and tail.**
- **Malignant potential: Main-duct IPMN > MCN > Branch-duct IPMN**

Okay, now that we've gone through all these cysts, here is a quick Board buzzword pop quiz. For each buzzword, name the cyst as fast as you can!

- Fish mouth ampulla
- Cluster of grapes
- Honeycombing
- Central scar
- Branched finger-like projection on cytology
- Mixed solid/cystic appearance

Finally, study Table 33-1 to bring it all together and check your answers to the buzzword quiz (this table is chock-a-block full of important tidbits—just know it cold!).

Table 33-1. THE MONEY TABLE!				
Variable	Mucinous Cystic Neoplasm	IPMNs	Serous Cystadenoma	Solid Pseudo-Papillary Neoplasm
Age	Middle-aged	Middle-aged to older	Older	Young! (< 40 yrs)
Gender	More in females	No gender bias!	More in females	Females (95%)
Imaging	98% body or tail (thick mucin)	"Fishmouth"; "cluster of grapes"	Microcystic or "honeycomb"; central scar	Mixed solid/cystic; in body/tail
Cytology	CEA > 192 Low amylase	CEA > 192 High amylase	Low CEA (< 0.5) + glycogen (cuboidal cells)	Low CEA Branching "finger-like" projections
Malignant Potential	Moderate	Low to high (depends…)	Way low	Moderate

Vignette 34: Was It the Bratwurst?

A 54-year-old man reports severe epigastric pain after eating bratwurst outside of Wrigley Field. He has eaten at this stand plenty of times as he's a long-time fan of the Chicago Cubs (who finally got that elusive World Series title in 2016) and has not had severe pain in the past; however, he reports a history of a milder but chronic epigastric discomfort radiating to the back for the past several months and diarrhea. He denies current or prior smoking, alcohol, or illicit drug use. On physical exam, he has epigastric tenderness to palpation, as well as parotid gland enlargement. Vital signs are temperature 98.3°F, blood pressure 115/85 mm Hg, heart rate 105 beats/minute, and oxygen saturation 100% on room air. Serum creatinine is 2.3 mg/dL. Liver tests are normal. Fecal elastase is 80 mcg/g. Tissue transglutaminase IgA and quantitative IgA are normal. An MRI of the abdomen is obtained (Figure 34-1).

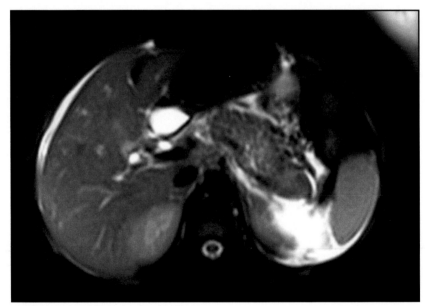

Figure 34-1. Axial T2 weighted MRI Image.

▶ *What is the diagnosis?*

▶ *What do you expect will be seen on biopsy of the pancreas?*

▶ *What other tests can help establish the diagnosis?*

▶ *What treatment should you recommend?*

Vignette 34: Answer

The MRI demonstrates a diffusely enlarged pancreas with featureless borders (ie "sausage pancreas") along with a low signal peripancreatic halo and severe peripancreatic inflammation. Sometimes, you can also see a thin, attenuated pancreatic duct. The main point here is that this pancreas actually looks like a bratwurst sausage including the skin (peripancreatic halo). These findings are highly suggestive of autoimmune pancreatitis (AIP). AIP can occur as a primary pancreatic disorder, or in association with IgG4-related autoimmune disorders in other organ systems (particularly the bile duct, salivary glands, kidneys, lungs, and thyroid gland). Pancreatic manifestations of AIP are nonspecific and range from chronic abdominal pain to recurrent acute or chronic pancreatitis, and a pancreatic mass. In this case, the patient also has evidence of chronic pancreatitis with pancreatic insufficiency (fecal elastase < 200 mcg/g). He also has signs suggestive of other organ involvement, including parotid gland enlargement (salivary gland involvement), and elevated creatinine (interstitial nephritis).

Serology can aid in the diagnosis of AIP. IgG4 normally accounts for 5% to 6% of total immunoglobulin G (ie < 140 mg/dL). An elevated serum IgG4 suggests AIP, particularly when the level is greater than twice the upper limit of normal. Unfortunately, serum IgG4 is not specific because pancreatic cancer can also cause elevated serum IgG4.

There are 2 histologic subtypes of AIP. Histological features of type 1 AIP (Figure 34-2) include an inflammatory periductal lymphoplasmacytic infiltrate often with IgG4-positive cells, acinar fibrosis, and obliterative phlebitis. In type 2 autoimmune pancreatitis, histology may demonstrate duct-centric pancreatitis or a granulocytic epithelial pancreatic duct lesion in the parenchyma with few IgG4-positive cells.

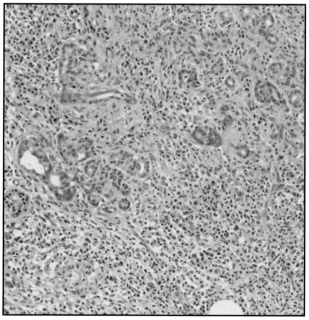

Figure 34-2. Type 1 autoimmune pancreatitis showing dense inflammatory infiltrate composed of lymphocytes, plasma cells, and eosinophils centered on pancreatic ducts. (Reprinted with permission from Vaidehi Avadhani, MD, Emory University.)

There are some clinical differences between these 2 subtypes of AIP. Type 1 AIP often involves other IgG4-related autoimmune disorders of other organ systems (bile duct, salivary glands, kidneys, lungs, and thyroid gland) and tends to present at a later age compared with type 2 AIP. Type 2 AIP occurs more commonly in association with IBD and has a lower relapse rate than type 1 AIP.

AIP typically responds to a course of steroids, which is the initial treatment for this condition. For patients who relapse after a course of steroids, various immunomodulators have been used for long-term therapy. By the way, the bratwurst had nothing to do with pain in this case. But now you can remember bratwurst (sausage) and autoimmune pancreatitis! Also, Dr. Karsan is a lifelong die-hard Cubs fan, so he insisted we include the Cubs somewhere in this book. Dr. Spiegel protested, but Dr. Karsan insisted. So there you have it.

Why Might This Be Tested? Autoimmune pancreatitis can cause symptoms of chronic pancreatitis or mimic pancreatic adenocarcinoma. You should know when to consider autoimmune pancreatitis in your differential, as the treatment and prognosis differ significantly from pancreatic adenocarcinoma and other causes of chronic pancreatitis.

Clinical Threshold Alert 1: Serum IgG4 is normally < 140 mg/dL. Serum IgG4 > 280 mg/dL is suggestive of type 1 autoimmune pancreatitis (BUT pancreatic cancer can also cause elevated IgG4 levels).

Clinical Threshold Alert 2: Fecal elastase < 200 mcg/g indicates pancreatic insufficiency

Here's the Point! 1

Abdominal pain or chronic pancreatitis + Sausage pancreas with peripancreatic halo and thin pancreatic duct on imaging = Autoimmune pancreatitis

Here's the Point! 2

Abnormal pancreas imaging + IgG4 related disorders + Periductal lymphoplasmacytic infiltrate = Type 1 autoimmune pancreatitis

Vignette 35: Pancreatic Mass

A 53-year-old man is seen in clinic for several months of a persistent aching epigastrium accompanied by an unintentional 20-lb weight loss. His wife recently noticed yellowing of his eyes and he has noticed dark urine and clay colored stools but no pruritis. He was previously in excellent health. He does not smoke cigarettes, drink alcohol, or use illicit drugs. Vital signs are normal. Liver tests show total bilirubin 3.1 mg/dL, alkaline phosphatase 455 U/L, AST 121 U/L, and ALT 101 U/L. A CT scan and then EUS (Figure 35-1) confirmed a 3-cm irregular heterogeneous mass in the head of the pancreas. An FNA is performed on the mass (Figure 35-2). Neither CT scan nor EUS demonstrates any malignant appearing adenopathy, distant metastases, or involvement of any vascular structures.

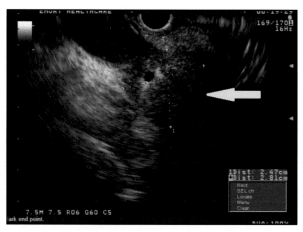

Figure 35-1. EUS image of pancreatic head mass. (Reprinted with permission from Jung Suh, MD, MPH, Atlanta Gastroenterology Associates.)

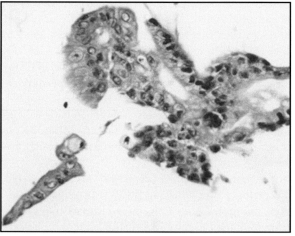

Figure 35-2. FNA of pancreatic mass.

▶ *What is the diagnosis?*

▶ *What should you recommend next?*

Vignette 35: Answer

The patient has pancreatic ductal adenocarcinoma. The term "pancreatic cancer" usually refers to ductal adenocarcinoma because it accounts for 85% of pancreatic neoplasms. The only potential cure for this otherwise highly lethal malignancy is surgical resection. In order to consider a patient for surgery, there must be no distant or nodal metastases or direct involvement of vascular structures (specifically the aorta, celiac artery, superior mesenteric artery, hepatic artery, and inferior vena cava). Also, the patient should be a reasonable operative candidate given the extent of surgery required. Some centers will consider surgery in patients with less than 180 degrees of vascular encasement by tumor after several months of chemotherapy +/− radiation. Such tumors are termed "borderline resectable" and the chemotherapy administered prior to surgery is termed neoadjuvant chemotherapy.

Preoperative jaundice was previously believed to increase the risk of postoperative complications, but randomized trials suggest that delaying surgery to decompress the bile duct actually increases the risk of postoperative complications. An ERCP prior to surgery may have been warranted if the patient had cholangitis, intractable pruritis, or if the operation was going to be delayed (eg neoadjuvant chemotherapy in a patient with borderline resectable pancreatic cancer). This patient has none of these features, so you should proceed directly to surgery without preoperative ERCP. We've seen too many cases of early pancreatic cancer turn into late pancreatic cancer because of unnecessary delay, sometimes spanning weeks or even months of planning, evaluating, testing, etc. Bottom line: If there's a mass in the head of the pancreas and no evidence of metastatic spread or vascular invasion, you've got to move on it—don't dillydally with lots of extra testing. That being said, you should counsel the patient, that even after successful surgery, his likelihood of surviving another 5 years is only 10% to 25%.

In this patient, the diagnosis was confirmed using FNA showing grouped malignant cells with enlarged basophilic nuclei with crowding. Thus, a finding of adenocarcinoma on FNA is highly specific for the diagnosis. However, a negative FNA does not rule out the diagnosis, particularly given the high pretest probability of cancer in this case. This has led some physicians to advocate proceeding directly to surgery without preoperative histologic confirmation in an otherwise healthy patient with a potentially resectable pancreatic mass. Think about it: If a 53-year-old has a mass in the head of the pancreas and you do an FNA that is "negative," are you even going to believe it? Are you just going to just reassure the patient and call off any further work-up? No chance. Pancreatic cancer is so deadly and can spread so fast that you've got to maintain a very low threshold for surgery (again, if no sign of spread, vascular invasion, and in the proper surgical candidate).

On the other hand, an aggressive approach could lead to unnecessary surgery in patients with pancreatic cancer mimickers, such as autoimmune pancreatitis or pancreatic sarcoidosis, but, in "real life," when you see a pancreatic mass in an older person, chances are (unfortunately) it is cancer, not autoimmune pancreatitis or something rare like sarcoid.

To make this a little bit personal, one of the authors had a family friend who was a 64-year-old, otherwise healthy man, who presented to his primary care physician (PCP) with epigastric pain without alarm signs or symptoms and without jaundice. The PCP diagnosed him with dyspepsia and started a proton pump inhibitor (PPI). He took the PPI for 4 weeks with little to no benefit. Next, the PCP tested him for *H. pylori*; the patient was positive and received treatment, but was no better weeks later. At this point in the story, it had been about 3 months since he first presented with epigastric pain. So, the PCP sent him to a GI doctor, who decided (appropriately) to do an upper endoscopy, which was negative. Now it had been 4 months since the pain started. The GI ordered a CT scan which promptly revealed the culprit: A mass in the uncinate process of the pancreas. There was no sign of vascular involvement, no nodal involvement, and no evidence of distant metastatic spread. Just like this case.

What happens next brings this vignette into sharp focus. The GI doctor decided to perform an ERCP with brushings—surgery was not presented as an option. The brushings came back negative, but the patient developed post-ERCP pancreatitis and was hospitalized for a week. After another considerable delay, he finally recovered from the pancreatitis but without definitive treatment for the mass; now it had been almost a half year since reporting epigastric pain to his PCP. Follow-up CT confirmed mass stability—there was still no sign of vascular involvement or distant spread. What did they do next? Well, he was sent to a "center of excellence" that decided to do an EUS with FNA. It was negative. Then, there was more hemming and hawing, more delay, more uncertainty for the patient and his family. The GI team decided to repeat the EUS with FNA, and this time the tissue returned positive for adenocarcinoma. It was finally time to operate. A week later he went to the OR and the surgeons found peritoneal studding, liver metastases, and vascular invasion. They closed without resecting anything. He died 2 months later, almost 10 months after initially presenting for care.

This case is instructive for several reasons. First, if an endoscopy is negative in an older person with persistent dyspepsia, as it was here, then it makes sense to proceed to imaging earlier than later. Depending on the nuances of the pain, some would go to CT even before an endoscopy, as supported by the latest American College of Gastroenterology dyspepsia guideline, which pragmatically emphasize that every patient has a different story and clinicians should remain wary of a pancreatic etiology of dyspepsia.

The other takeaway from this case is that when a pancreatic mass is found, it's like a ticking time bomb. The patient doesn't have much time. You don't have much time. In fact, even with a favorable appearing CT scan, the tumor may already have spread but remains below the radar. You should not do an ERCP with brushings at this point. In this case, it was diagnostically useless and, worse, caused avoidable suffering and delay. Even doing EUS with FNA is controversial, as we've discussed. Some surgeons insist on knowing the tissue results before they operate, arguing that it supports a more informed conversation with the patient before the surgery (and this makes sense, so long as they'll still operate with a negative FNA). Finally, we'll never know if this patient would have survived had surgery occurred months (or even weeks) earlier, but by the time the surgeons got in… it was too late.

When you see a pancreatic mass, move on it. Don't delay.

Why Might This Be Tested? Pancreatic ductal adenocarcinoma is the fourth leading cause of cancer related death in the United States. Because surgical resection is the only potential cure, you should know when to promptly proceed with an operation. On the other hand, pancreatic surgery is associated with substantial morbidity, so you should also know when an operation is unlikely to benefit the patient.

Here's the Point!

> **Pancreatic cancer + Jaundice + Good operative candidate, no distant or nodal metastases, no direct vascular involvement = Proceed to surgical resection**

Vignette 36: Managing Time

A 60-year-old woman with a 5-cm mass in the head of the pancreas undergoes EUS with FNA and is diagnosed as having unresectable pancreatic cancer due to complete encasement of the celiac and superior mesenteric arteries. There are no distant metastases. The patient is otherwise healthy without other comorbid conditions. She does not report pruritis and has no signs of cholangitis. Her oncologist prognosticates that with chemotherapy and radiation, her survival should exceed 6 months.

Liver tests show total bilirubin 12 mg/dL, alkaline phosphatase 800 U/L, AST 180 U/L, and ALT 200 U/L.

▶ *How should you manage this patient's jaundice?*

Vignette 36: Answer

There is a saying that "jaundice never kills anyone." It's not a very empathetic dictum, but it is true nonetheless—jaundice, unto itself, does not cause mortality. Thus, the concept of "palliating jaundice" is not accurate. In contrast, palliation applies to pain, pruritis (which can be a maddening symptom), and of course, cholangitis. In this case, the patient has jaundice without pruritis or signs of cholangitis and may be considered a "cosmetic" issue. Nonetheless, if the malignant biliary obstruction is not managed now, then it will be a matter of time before she develops complications; it is reasonable to manage the obstruction now.

There are 3 methods of managing surgically unresectable malignant biliary obstruction—surgical bypass (hepaticojejunostomy), percutaneous drainage, and endoscopic decompression (ERCP with stent placement). Surgery and percutaneous drainage are associated with a higher risk of complications and a decreased quality of life when compared to the endoscopic approach. Therefore, endoscopic decompression is the preferred strategy for palliating malignant biliary obstruction.

For Board review purposes, you don't need to know every intimate detail about stent composition, diameter, length, etc. However, you should know when to place a plastic vs a self-expandable metallic stent (SEMS) in patients with unresectable malignant obstructive jaundice. Plastic stents are cheaper and easier to remove than SEMS. However, even the larger 10 to 11.5 French (approximately 4 mm) plastic stents tend to occlude within 4 to 5 months, mandating repeat ERCP procedures. SEMS are more expensive, but remain patent a lot longer than plastic stents predominantly due to their larger diameter (10 mm). SEMS are cost effective compared to plastic stents if a patient's anticipated survival is greater than 3 months, due to reduced number of ERCP procedures.

This patient has an anticipated survival greater than 3 months, so you should go with metal. That is, the preferred method of palliating jaundice in this case is to perform an ERCP and place a SEMS in the bile duct. It is probably worth knowing that if you plan to deploy the proximal end of the SEMS above the cystic duct in a patient with an intact gallbladder, you should choose an uncovered SEMS to reduce risk of occluding the cystic duct and causing cholecystitis. Similarly, if you plan to deploy the proximal end of the SEMS within the intrahepatic duct, then you should choose an uncovered SEMS to avoid "jailing off" bile flow from one lobe of the liver. Covered SEMS have their own inherent advantages, such as allowing less tumor ingrowth and are typically easier to remove than the uncovered SEMS.

Percutaneous biliary drainage does have a role as a salvage therapy if endoscopic stenting is unsuccessful (eg duodenal obstruction that does not permit passage of the duodenoscope) or obstruction is primarily within the intrahepatic bile ducts.

Clinical Threshold Alert: 3 French = 1 mm; the largest plastic biliary stent is 11.5 French (~4 mm); the largest biliary SEMS are 10 mm in diameter.

Here's the Point!

**Unresectable malignant jaundice + Anticipated survival > 3 months =
Perform ERCP and place a metal stent**

Vignette 37: Change the Bulb

An 80-year-old man with 30-lb weight loss and abdominal pain is found to have a 6-cm mass in the head of the pancreas, with liver metastases, peripancreatic adenopathy and invasion of the celiac artery and superior mesenteric artery. His medical history includes coronary artery disease, COPD, end stage renal disease requiring hemodialysis, and poorly controlled diabetes. An upper endoscopy is performed prior to the planned EUS, and reveals obstruction at the junction of the bulb and second portion of the duodenum from tumor invasion. Duodenal biopsies confirm the diagnosis of adenocarcinoma. Liver tests show total bilirubin 10 mg/dL, alkaline phosphatase 600 U/L, AST 130 U/L, and ALT 150 U/L. He is evaluated by an oncologist and is not considered a candidate for systemic chemotherapy due to his poor performance status.

▶ *How should you palliate this patient's enteral obstruction?*

Vignette 37: Answer

The 2 options for palliating malignant gastroduodenal obstruction are surgical gastrojejunostomy and upper endoscopy with enteral stent placement. Although surgery provides more durable palliation of gastroduodenal obstruction, enteral stents are cheaper, less invasive, and provide quicker palliation. Gastrojejunostomy can be considered in patients who are reasonable operative candidates and have an anticipated life expectancy > 6 months.

This patient with multiple comorbid conditions and poor performance status should receive an enteral stent. Prior to placing the enteral stent, he should undergo decompression of obstructive jaundice because the stent scaffolding can make bile duct cannulation challenging. In this case, since the duodenoscope cannot traverse the duodenal sweep, he should undergo percutaneous biliary drainage. As an aside, some centers perform EUS-guided biliary drainage in this setting to avoid putting the patient through an additional percutaneous drainage procedure. Because this technique is not widely performed, it is not critical for Board review purposes to choose between EUS-guided biliary drainage and percutaneous drainage.

Following external biliary drain placement, bile flows into an external bag attached to the drain. Patients may find this to negatively impact their quality of life, in which case the radiologist can internalize the drain later (ie advance the drainage tube antegrade past the major papilla so that bile is directed into the duodenum). Even with an internalized drain, the patient is still left with an external catheter. This too can later be converted to an internal stent placed either antegrade by the radiologist or retrograde by the endoscopist through the enteral stent scaffolding if needed.

Here's the Point! 1

Malignant gastroduodenal obstruction + Life expectancy < 6 months = Place an uncovered metal enteral stent

Here's the Point! 2

Malignant obstructive jaundice + Malignant gastroduodenal obstruction = Perform biliary decompression before placing an enteral stent

Vignettes 38-45: Stoned

Okay, you're about to get stoned. In this mini quiz, we first describe a brief one-liner patient, and then you tell us what type of gallstone the patient is most likely to develop. That's it, just name the type of stone. (Hint: There are 3 major types of gallstones—(1) cholesterol; (2) black pigment or bilirubin; and (3) brown pigment or mixed. So you have nearly a 1 in 3 chance to get these right!)

38.   A young African American with longstanding anemia and no spleen.

39.   An alcoholic with esophageal varices and encephalopathy.

40.   A woman who is 24-weeks pregnant.

41.   An Asian patient with innumerable stones piled up the CBD and left hepatic duct, but none in the gallbladder.

42.   A patient with rapid weight loss from a "crash diet."

43.   A patient with neurofibromatosis, a pancreatic tumor, diarrhea, and diabetes.

44.   A patient on longstanding total parenteral nutrition (TPN).

45.   A patient with sepsis on ceftriaxone.

Vignette 38-45: Answers

Because gallstones are common, occurring in 10% to 15% of people in the developed world, you will frequently encounter them in clinical practice. As we mentioned earlier, there are 3 major types of gallstones: (1) cholesterol; (2) black pigment or bilirubin; and (3) brown pigment or mixed.

Cholesterol stones are by far the most prevalent, accounting for more than 80% of gallstones. They occur when the bile contains excess cholesterol and too little bile salts, leading to supersaturation of cholesterol and precipitation out of solution, eventually forming sludge or, when organized and hard, a yellow-green stone. Technically speaking, a cholesterol stone must be composed of at least 80% cholesterol. Risk factors for cholesterol stones include anything that can slow motility of the gallbladder, cause cholestasis, reduce the concentration of bile salts or increase the concentration of cholesterol (more below).

In contrast, bilirubin stones, which are also called black pigment stones (Figure 38-1) form when bile is supersaturated with insoluble bilirubin pigment and calcium phosphate salts. These stones contain less than 20% cholesterol. Anything that releases excess bilirubin—most notably hemolytic anemias—can lead to pigment stones forming in the biliary system.

Mixed stones are just that—a combination of cholesterol, calcium salts, bilirubin, and other bile pigments like calcium bilirubinate, calcium palmitate, and calcium stearate. Basically, they contain the whole kitchen sink. Mixed stones, also called brown pigment stones (Figure 38-2), technically contain between 20% and 80% cholesterol. They may form in the setting of recurrent cholangitis, where bacteria trapped in the biliary system release β-glucuronidase from injured hepatocytes and from their own cell walls. This, in turn, hydrolyzes bilirubin glucuronides and leads to excess unconjugated bilirubin in the bile.

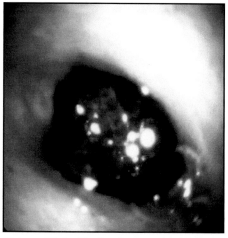

Figure 38-1. Black pigment stone seen on choledochoscopy. (Reprinted with permission from Jung Suh, MD, MPH, Atlanta Gastroenterology Associates.)

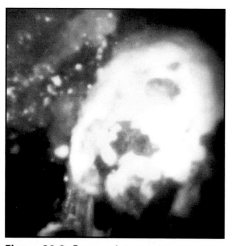

Figure 38-2. Brown pigment stone seen on choledochoscopy. (Reprinted with permission from Nandhakumar Kanagarajan, MD, Atlanta Gastroenterology Associates.)

Okay, with that background, this should be pretty easy:

38.   This is a patient with sickle cell anemia who is predisposed to bilirubin or black pigment stones from hemolytic anemia. The same would occur with, say, hereditary spherocytosis.

39.   This is a patient with cirrhosis and therefore has a variety of reasons to have an increased rate of gallstone formation. Remember that there is decreased production of bile salts by the liver in cirrhotics, who can also experience a hemolytic anemia from fragile cell walls. So, you can see spiculated red blood cells such as echinocytes (burr cells) and acanthocytes (spur cells) in addition to target cells in liver disease. This all leads to formation of predominantly bilirubin or black pigment stones in patients with chronic liver disease. Moreover, cirrhotics also have an elevated estrogen level that increases the rate of stone formation.

40.   Pregnant women are at risk of developing cholesterol stones from estrogen-induced biliary hypokinesis and cholestasis, coupled with reduced bile acid secretion from progesterone.

41.   This is recurrent pyogenic cholangitis (see earlier in book). Recall that these patients have brown pigment stones, but they're not typically in the gallbladder; instead, they're everywhere but the gallbladder.

42.   Rapid weight loss (eg from a "crash diet") can generate cholesterol stones. There is evidence that increasing the relative fat content in the diet can help reduce gallstone formation during planned aggressive weight loss. Some also use ursodeoxycholic acid (UCDA), a bile acid, to prevent stone formation with some success during periods of planned weight loss. While we're on the topic of UCDA, in what other conditions is it effective? Does it work for primary biliary cholangitis (PBC)? How about for primary sclerosing cholangitis (PSC)? Is it helpful in recurrent pyogenic cholangitis? What about for cholestasis of cystic fibrosis? Noodle on that for a bit. We'll give you the answers soon.

43.   This patient has a somatostatinoma. Did you figure that out? If so, kudos to you! Somatostatinoma is associated with neurofibromatosis—an important association to remember for Board review. It causes diarrhea, diabetes, and biliary dyskinesia with cholesterol gallstone formation. Stay tuned for more on somatostatinoma later in the book.

44.   Patients on TPN can develop bile stasis due to lack of enteral feeds. This predisposes to cholesterol stones.

45. This patient received ceftriaxone which can reach high concentrations in bile (100 to 200 times its serum concentration). This can lead to crystal formation with calcium concretions bound to ceftriaxone itself. This is a special kind of stone unique to ceftriaxone.

There are a bunch of risk factors for gallstones you should know about. We've covered most of them in the vignettes, but here is a table to remind you of the predisposing conditions and clues to look for:

Table 45-1.		
RISK FACTORS FOR GALLSTONES		
Risk Factor	*Clues in Question Stem*	*Type of Stone*
High estrogen	• Pregnant • Estrogen replacement therapy • Female patient (risk unto itself)	Cholesterol
Biliary dyskinesia	• Fasting • On TPN • Crash diet • Somatostatinoma (diarrhea, diabetes, pancreatic mass, neurofibromatosis)	Cholesterol
Obesity	• Self-evident…	Cholesterol
Hemolysis	• Cirrhosis • Sickle cell anemia • Hereditary spherocytosis	Bilirubin or black pigment stones
Recurrent pyogenic cholangitis	• From Asia • **No** gallstones • Innumerable stones in CBD and hepatic ducts—left hepatic duct in particular	Mixed or brown pigment stones

Oh, right, those UDCA questions. Here are the answers to that little pop quiz:

Weight loss → Yes; cholesterol stones from biliary dyskinesia may respond to UDCA.
PBC → Yes; UDCA can help reduce disease progression.
PSC → No; UDCA does not reduce disease progression.
Recurrent pyogenic cholangitis → No; mixed stones not dissolvable by UDCA.
Cholestasis of cystic fibrosis → Probably.

Vignette 46: A 3D Experience at DDW

A 50-year-old man is evaluated for a 6-month history of large volume, watery diarrhea that often awakens him at night. He has lost 20 lb in the last 6 months. He was recently diagnosed with diabetes. He also complains of a painful, pruritic rash on his face and extremities (Figure 46-1). He takes insulin for his diabetes but does not take any other medications. He does not smoke cigarettes, drink alcohol, or use illicit drugs. Complete blood count, serum chemistry and liver tests are normal. EGD with duodenal biopsies is normal. Colonoscopy with random biopsies is also normal.

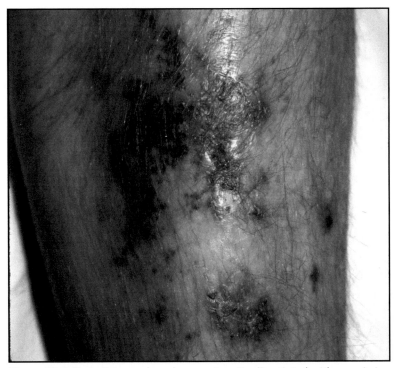

Figure 46-1. Necrotizing rash on lower extremity. (Reprinted with permission from Robert A. Swerlick, MD, Emory University.)

▶ *What is the diagnosis?*

▶ *What is this rash called?*

Vignette 46: Answer

This patient has the classic "3D" triad of glucagonoma—"Diarrhea (secretory), Dermatitis, and Diabetes." There is typically weight loss associated with this tumor. So if you need an aid to remember, then think "DDW" (ie "Digestive Disease Week"), but here it stands for "Diabetes," "Dermatitis," and "Weight Loss" (okay, plus "Diarrhea" for the third "D," but that would be "DDDW"). The classic rash is called necrolytic migratory erythema (NME) and is characterized by painful pruritic erythematous papules and plaques on the face, perineum, and extremities that coalesce and then develop central clearing with blistering, crusting, and scaling at the borders. NME is not pathognomonic for glucagonoma since it can also occur in other GI conditions like celiac disease, IBD, and cystic fibrosis (all of which can also cause diarrhea). However, when this rash is associated with recent onset of diabetes and other signs like cheilosis, you should strongly suspect a glucagonoma. For Board review purposes, always strongly suspect a glucagonoma.

Unlike pancreatic adenocarcinoma, glucagonomas arise from the endocrine cells of the pancreas (ie they are a type of pancreatic neuroendocrine tumor). As the name suggests, these tumors release glucagon so serum glucagon levels should be elevated. Etiologies associated with physiologic stress can also mildly elevate serum glucagon levels (eg sepsis, hypoglycemia, fasting, acute pancreatitis, etc). But a serum glucagon >500 pg/mL is much more suggestive of a glucaganoma than an alternative diagnosis. Glucagonomas tend to be large at initial presentation, and are usually detected on cross-sectional imaging (CT scan or MRI). Most patients have metastatic disease at diagnosis. CT or ultrasound-guided biopsy can establish the diagnosis in patients with liver metastases. In patients with nonmetastatic disease, EUS-FNA can provide histologic confirmation. Hepatic resection is an option for patients with limited liver metastases confined to a single lobe. If surgery is not an option, somatostatin analogs like octreotide can provide symptomatic relief.

Why Might This Be Tested? Skin manifestations of GI conditions, like the NME rash of glucagonoma are important for Board review.

Clinical Threshold Alert: Serum glucagon >500 pg/mL is suggestive of a glucagonoma.

Here's the Point!

Diarrhea + Diabetes + NME rash = Glucagonoma

Vignette 47: A Very Important Patient (VIP)

A 40-year-old woman undergoes evaluation for several months of large volume diarrhea that wakes her up from sleep. She has had 2 hospitalizations for dehydration due to diarrhea. She also complains of flushing. On examination, the patient appears comfortable. Her abdomen is soft and not tender to palpation. Complete blood count and liver tests are normal. Serum chemistry is normal except for serum potassium of 2.5 mEq/L and serum chloride of 95 mmol/L. Stool sodium is 100 mmol/L and stool potassium is 30 mmol/L. Upper endoscopy with duodenal biopsies and colonoscopy with random biopsies are normal. There is a 3.5-cm, well-defined, round hypoechoic hypervascular mass on CT scan in the tail of the pancreas.

▶ *What's the diagnosis?*

▶ *How do you interpret her stool electrolytes?*

Vignette 47: Answer

A mass in the pancreas always raises concern for pancreatic adenocarcinoma, and this diagnosis certainly needs to be ruled out. That being said, pancreatic adenocarcinomas tend to appear irregular and heterogeneous. This patient has a round, well-defined, hypervascular, solid pancreatic mass, which is more suggestive of a pancreatic neuroendocrine tumor (PNET).

PNETs can be nonfunctional or functional. Functional PNETs cause symptoms due to excess release of a dominant hormone. Examples are insulinoma, glucagonoma, gastrinoma, somatostatinoma, functional carcinoids and VIPoma. VIPoma is a rare PNET associated with a characteristic "WDHA syndrome" (Watery Diarrhea, Hypokalemia, Achlorhydria). VIPomas typically occur in the tail of the pancreas, and can also cause flushing. You should suspect a VIPoma in this patient with all the characteristic features. Functional carcinoid tumors can also cause flushing and secretory diarrhea, but profound hypochlorhydria/achlorhydria would be unusual—a key point to differentiate carcinoid from VIPoma. Serum VIP is typically > 75 pg/mL in patients with VIPoma. In patients with metastatic disease, octreotide can provide symptomatic relief.

By the way, you should know how to interpret stool electrolytes. We cover this in the original *Acing* book, but here's a refresher: Stool osmolar gap = 290 − 2 (stool sodium + stool potassium). Stool osmolar gap < 50 mOsm/kg suggests a secretory diarrhea, while osmolar gap > 50 mOsm/kg (and more often > 125) suggests osmotic diarrhea. This patient's stool osmolar gap is 290 − 2 (100 + 30) = 30 mOsm/kg, which is consistent with a secretory diarrhea.

While we are on the topic of round solid masses in the pancreas, you should also consider the possibility of metastases to the pancreas, which can present as a solitary lesion or with multiple pancreatic lesions. Pancreatic metastases are uncommon and account for only 2% to 5% of pancreatic malignancies. Renal cell carcinoma is the most common malignancy that metastasizes to the pancreas, followed by melanoma. Nice facts to remember because they'll be coming back at 'ya in the "Crunch-Time" Self-Test later in the book.

Why Might This Be Tested? Although VIPoma is rare, it presents with a characteristic clinical "WDHA syndrome" that connects the pancreas to the GI lumen (diarrhea). That makes VIPoma an excellent topic for GI Board review.

Clinical Threshold Alert 1: Serum VIP is > 75 pg/mL in VIPoma.

Clinical Threshold Alert 2: Stool osmolar gap = 290 − 2 (stool sodium + stool potassium)
Stool osmolar gap < 50 mOsm/kg → Secretory diarrhea
Stool osmolar gap > 50 mOsm/kg → Osmotic diarrhea

Here's the Point!

> **Round solid mass in pancreatic tail + WDHA syndrome = VIPoma**

Vignette 48: Pour Some Sugar on Me

A 55-year-old woman has repeated episodes of symptomatic hypoglycemia that improves with administration of glucose. She is constantly craving sugar, but does not carry a diagnosis of diabetes. She has also noted a milky discharge from her breasts over the past few months. Her medical history is significant for a parathyroid adenoma that was resected several years ago. She does not smoke cigarettes, drink alcohol, or use any illicit drugs. She vaguely recalls that her father had a "pancreas problem," and her paternal grandfather had a brain tumor that was removed. During a monitored prolonged fast, symptoms occur after 24 hours. At that time, pertinent laboratory studies are serum glucose 35 mg/dL, serum C-peptide 0.4 nmol/L, undetectable serum sulfonylurea and a negative insulin antibody screen. Serum calcium is 11.2 mg/dL.

▶ *What's the diagnosis?*

▶ *What risk factor does she have for this diagnosis?*

Vignette 48: Answer

This patient has an insulinoma. This rare functional pancreatic neuroendocrine tumor presents with a characteristic symptom pattern due to excessive insulin termed "Whipple's triad" (symptoms of hypoglycemia + low plasma glucose during symptoms + relief of symptoms with administration of glucose). You can confirm the diagnosis by performing a 72-hour fast and obtaining laboratory studies when symptoms occur. By definition, the patient must have hypoglycemia when symptoms occur. So, they literally need to pour sugar into their bodies and hence the title of this vignette. That also allows for a nice Def Leppard reference for those fans of 80s hair bands. By the way, Def Leppard's earlier *Pyromania* album has to be considered one of the best of all time.

Surreptitious insulin or sulfonylurea use can also cause hypoglycemia. A sulfonylurea blood screen excluded surreptitious sulfonylurea use in this case. You can rule out hypoglycemia due to insulin by checking a serum C-peptide level at the end of the fast. Recall that C-peptide is a component of endogeneous insulin, but is not present in commercially available insulin preparations. If hypoglycemia is due to surreptitious insulin, serum C-peptide will be low (<0.2 nmol/L). Here, the C-peptide level was high which rules out factitious hypoglycemia from exogenous insulin. Autoimmune insulin hypoglycemia is another rare syndrome that can also cause symptomatic hypoglycemia with an elevated C-peptide, but her insulin antibody screen was negative, which rules that out too. So, this patient's diagnosis is insulinoma. The next step is to localize the tumor with imaging studies and resect if feasible.

Not only does this patient have an insulinoma, but you should suspect autosomal dominant multiple endocrine neoplasia-1 (MEN-1) syndrome in this patient with a pancreatic neuroendocrine tumor (insulinoma) who also has a pituitary adenoma (prolactinoma causing galactorrhea) and parathyroid adenoma causing hypercalcemia. The MEN-1 gene on chromosome 11 encodes a tumor suppressor protein called menin. Patients with MEN-1 mutations have an increased risk of developing the "3Ps" (**P**arathyroid adenomas, **P**ituitary adenomas, and **P**ancreatic neuroendocrine tumors). Of patients with MEN-1, 80% to 100% develop PNETs. For GI Board review, you should also know the other inherited conditions that increase risk of PNETs (Table 48-1).

Table 48-1.			
INHERITED RISK FACTORS FOR PNET. THIS TABLE IS FULL OF GOLDEN NUGGETS. MINE THE GOLD NOW, YOU'LL THANK US LATER.			
Disorder	*Inheritance*	*Types of PNETs (% incidence)*	*Other features*
MEN-1	Autosomal dominant	All (80% to 100%)	• Parathyroid tumors • Pituitary tumors
von Hippel-Lindau	Autosomal dominant	All (20%)	• Pheochromocytoma • Hemangioblastoma • Renal cell carcinoma
NF-1	Autosomal dominant	Somatostatinoma (10%)	• Pheochromocytoma • Café au lait spots • Neurofibromas
Tuberous sclerosis	Autosomal dominant	Insulinoma (1%)	• Rhabdomyoma • Angiomyolipoma • Renal cysts

Here's the Point! 1

Parathyroid adenoma + Pituitary adenoma + Pancreatic neuroendocrine tumor (3 Ps) = MEN-1

Here's the Point! 2

Symptomatic hypoglycemia with fasting in a nondiabetic + Elevated C-peptide = Insulinoma

Vignette 49: Stony River

A 50-year-old woman presents with several months of watery diarrhea and right upper quadrant discomfort. The abdominal discomfort typically occurs after a heavy meal and lasts about 30 minutes before spontaneous resolution. The watery diarrhea occurs postpandially also with large volume and oily stools. She was recently diagnosed with diabetes mellitus. On physical examination, you note soft, fleshy nodules throughout the body (Figure 49-1). There are also several uniform brown macules throughout her body. Complete blood count, serum chemistry, and liver tests are normal. A CT scan of the abdomen is obtained and demonstrates several gallstones as well as a 5-cm uniform, round pancreatic head mass. Several uniform round masses are also present throughout the liver.

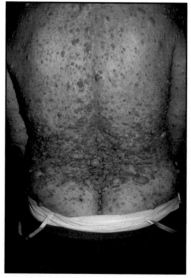

Figure 49-1. Soft, nontender nodules on back. (Reprinted with permission from Robert A. Swerlick, MD, Emory University.)

▶ *What's going on here?*

Vignette 49: Answer

This patient has a combination of gallstones and watery, flowing diarrhea—the "stony river" of somatostatinoma. There are several clues to note here. A uniform round pancreatic mass is more suggestive of a pancreatic neuroendocrine tumor than an adenocarcinoma. The patient presents with the classic somatostatinoma syndrome triad of diarrhea, diabetes, and gallstones (recall from Vignette 43). Also, somatostatinomas can occur as the pancreatic endocrine tumor in the MEN-1 syndrome. Moreover, they are frequently associated with neurofibromatosis-1 (NF-1). This woman has the characteristic findings of NF-1 including neurofibromas (Figure 49-1) and café-au-lait spots (uniform brown macules). Those are important tidbits to remember.

Somatostatinomas are rare neuroendocrine tumors that can occur in the duodenum and in the pancreas. In the duodenum, somatostatinomas tend not to cause the somatostatinoma syndrome as they usually are small and less than 3 cm at diagnosis. However, when somatostatinomas are found in the pancreas, they average 5 cm and release excessive amounts of inhibitory hormone, producing the somatostatinoma syndrome. Somatostatin inhibits cholecystokinin, resulting in decreased gallbladder contractility and formation of gallstones due to stasis. Cholecystokinin inhibition also decreases pancreatic enzyme secretion, leading to malabsorptive diarrhea. Finally, somatostatin inhibits insulin release, which predisposes to diabetes mellitus. Unfortunately, three-fourths of somatostatinomas are metastatic at diagnosis as is the case with this patient, especially when found in the pancreas. Somewhat paradoxically, the somatostatin analog octreotide can provide symptomatic relief in patients with metastatic somatostatinomas.

Why Might This Be Tested? Somatostatinomas are rare, but they present with a characteristic clinical syndrome and can be associated with MEN-1 and NF-1. You know how important these syndromes are!

Here's the Point!

Round pancreatic mass + Diarrhea, gallstones, diabetes = Somatostatinoma

Vignette 50: Rest Easy

A 54-year-old man is seen in consultation for persistent dyspepsia. He was tested for *H. pylori* with the stool antigen, which was negative. He then took a proton pump inhibitor for 8 weeks without any relief in symptoms. He has not lost weight, and has not noticed blood in his stool. He had a cholecystectomy several years ago for symptomatic cholelithiasis. Vital signs are temperature 98.4°F, blood pressure 120/80 mm Hg, pulse 85 beats/minute, and oxygen saturation 100% on room air. On physical exam, there is mild tenderness in the epigastrium. Complete blood count, liver tests, and serum chemistries are normal. An upper endoscopy is performed. The lesion in Figure 50-1 is seen in the antrum.

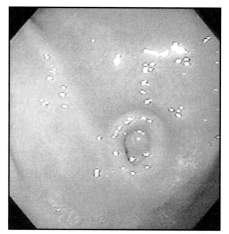

Figure 50-1. Bump in the antrum. (Reprinted with permission from Firas H. Al-Kawas, MD, FACP, FACG.)

▶ *What's the diagnosis?*

Vignette 50: Answer

This is ectopic pancreatic tissue also called a "pancreatic rest." You can rest easy, because this is just a rest (and the question is easy, too). The patient can also be restful, because he's just full of rest, and now you know the rest of the story. Okay, enough…

What differentiates a pancreatic rest from other subepithelial lesions on endoscopy is the presence of central umbilication, which corresponds to a draining duct. This image looks like a tiny volcano with a crater at the top. Pancreatic rests are histologically normal pancreatic tissue and usually require no intervention. However, they can occasionally ulcerate and bleed or grow large enough to cause gastric outlet obstruction, in which case, resection is recommended. But in this case, all looks fine—the patient can rest easy.

For Board review, you generally don't have to know too much about EUS image interpretation. The exception is EUS of gastric subepithelial lesions. Know that the layers of the stomach from superficial to deep are the mucosa, muscularis mucosa, submucosa, muscularis propria, and the serosa. On endoscopic ultrasound, the muscle layers appear dark while the mucosa and submucosa appear relatively bright. Lesions that are darker than the muscle layers are hypoechoic. Lesions that are brighter than the mucosa or submucosa are hyperechoic. If the echogenicity is equivalent to the involved layer, then the lesion is isoechoic. A dark black lesion is termed anechoic, and indicates that it is filled with fluid (like blood from varices or cystic fluid). The layer of origin and echogenicity allow you to differentiate subepithelial lesions on EUS. For instance, a pancreatic rest typically arises from submucosa and is relatively hypoechoic (Figure 50-2). A carcinoid tumor or a granular cell tumor could also have a similar appearance. On the other hand, a gastrointestinal stromal tumor (GIST) or a leiomyoma would arise from a muscle layer and not the submucosa. Although a lipoma arises from the submucosa, it is hyperechoic, whereas a pancreatic rest is relatively hypoechoic.

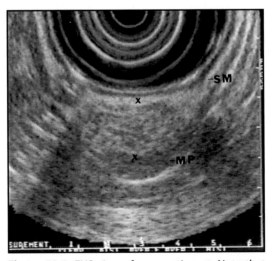

Figure 50-2. EUS view of pancreatic rest. Note that the lesion arises from the submusosa (SM) and does not invade the muscularis propria (MP). (Reprinted with permission from Firas H. Al-Kawas, MD, FACP, FACG.)

Table 50-1.		
GASTRIC SUB-EPITHELIAL LESIONS (SEE ORIGINAL ACING BOOK FOR MUCH MORE ON THESE TUMORS)		
EUS Appearance	*Origin = Third layer (submucosa)*	*Origin = Second or Fourth layer (muscularis mucosa or muscularis propria)*
Anechoic	• Duplication cyst • Varices	
Hypoechoic	• Carcinoid • Granular cell tumor • Pancreatic rest	• GI stromal tumor (GIST) • Leiomyoma • Leiomyosarcoma
Hyperechoic	Lipoma	
Isoechoic	Carcinoid	

Vignette 51: Duct, Duct, Goose

An 18-year-old Japanese woman is seen in clinic for several years of chronic vague right upper quadrant discomfort. She has no other medical problems. She has no weight loss or blood in her stool. She drinks a moderate quantity of alcohol on occasion. She does not smoke cigarettes or use any illicit drugs. Vital signs are temperature 98.4°F, blood pressure 100/60 mm Hg, pulse 70 beats/minute, and oxygen saturation 100% on room air. On physical examination, her abdomen is soft and nontender to palpation. Complete blood count, serum chemistry, and liver tests are normal. A right upper quadrant ultrasound reveals no gallstones, but the common bile duct is dilated to 14 mm. Subsequently, an ERCP is performed (shown below in Figure 51-1).

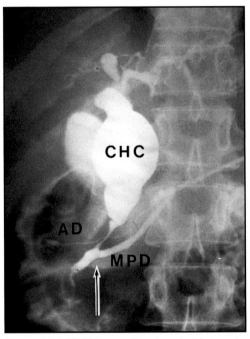

Figure 51-1. ERCP image. (Reprinted with permission from Anthony J. DiMarino Jr, MD and Stanley B. Benjamin, MD.)

► *What are the findings on this ERCP?*

► *How should you manage this finding?*

Vignette 51: Answer

The patient has 2 related findings on ERCP. The first is a type I biliary cyst (labeled CHC in Figure 51-1), which is a fusiform dilation of the extrahepatic bile duct. The second finding is an abnormal panc-bil junction (arrow in Figure 51-1) or APBJ. We briefly covered both entities in the "ERCP Extravaganza" earlier in the book, but we'll describe them in a bit more detail here.

In patients with an APBJ, the common bile duct and the main pancreatic duct (MPD in Figure 51-1) fuse outside the duodenal wall, and a long, common channel leads to the duodenal lumen. Of note, some patients may have an accessory pancreatic duct of Santorini (AD in Figure 51-1) draining separately into the duodenum via the minor duodenal papilla. An APBJ is present in about 70% of patients with type I biliary cysts. A possible explanation for the association between APBJ and biliary cysts is that a long common channel predisposes to reflux of pancreatic juices into the biliary tree. Pancreatic juices damage the biliary epithelium, resulting in biliary cyst formation. Biliary cysts are more common in women, and the incidence is highest among Asians (including Japanese).

The main clinical significance of these findings is that biliary cysts predispose to cholangio-carcinoma, especially if the patient also has an APBJ. An APBJ predisposes to gallbladder cancer, even in patients without biliary cysts. Since this patient with an APBJ and type I biliary cyst is otherwise young and healthy, you should recommend surgery to reduce her risk of developing biliary and gallbladder cancer. Specifically, she should undergo complete excision of the extrahepatic bile duct as well as a cholecystectomy. Following excision biliary drainage is re-established by anastomosing the intrahepatic biliary system to the small intestine (typically via Roux-en-Y hepaticojejunostomy). Table 51-1 outlines the management of biliary cysts.

What if a patient has an APBJ but doesn't have bile duct dilation or biliary cysts? Are they in the clear? No, they're not. There is still a risk of developing gallbladder cancer and a cholecystectomy is still recommended.

Why Might This Be Tested? Biliary cysts and APBJ provide an excellent opportunity to test your ERCP clinical knowledge. More importantly, you can significantly impact a patient's risk of developing 2 highly lethal cancers by recognizing and appropriately treating these findings.

Table 51-1.			
BILIARY CYSTS			
Cyst type	*Description*	*Cancer Risk*	*Management*
I	Fusiform extrahepatic bile duct dilation	Highest	Complete extrahepatic bile duct resection
II	Diverticula that communicate with the common bile duct through a narrow stalk	Lower	Simple excision of diverticulum
III	Cystic dilation of the intraduodenal portion of the common bile duct (choledochocele)	Lowest	Endoscopic sphincterotomy if young or symptomatic +/– cyst excision
IV	Multiple extrahepatic bile duct cysts +/– intrahepatic bile duct cysts	Highest	Complete extrahepatic bile duct resection (+/– partial hepatectomy if intrahepatic cysts)
V	Multiple intrahepatic bile duct cysts (Caroli disease)	High	Challenging and variable (from supportive care to liver transplantation)

Here's the Point! 1

In type I biliary cysts, only the extrahepatic bile duct is dilated; however, when there is extrahepatic biliary obstruction both the extrahepatic and intrahepatic bile ducts are dilated.

Here's the Point! 2

Asian woman + Fusion of bile duct and pancreatic duct outside duodenum + Long common channel = APBJ (increases risk of gallbladder cancer)

Vignette 52: Give Me a Ring

A 21-year-old man presents with several months of postprandial abdominal pain, nausea, vomiting, and unintentional 10-lb weight loss. Vital signs are temperature 98.8°F, blood pressure 110/80 mm Hg, pulse 80 beats/minute, and oxygen saturation 99% on room air. On physical exam, there is a succussion splash in the epigastric region but no tenderness to palpation. Complete blood count, serum chemistry, and liver enzymes are normal. An abdominal X-ray is obtained and demonstrates a dilated stomach and duodenal bulb with paucity of gas in the distal duodenum. An EGD is performed and the scope is advanced to the second portion of the duodenum. There is a large volume of clear liquid in the stomach and duodenal bulb, and an extrinsic compression distal to the major papilla. A CT scan with contrast is obtained (shown below in Figure 52-1).

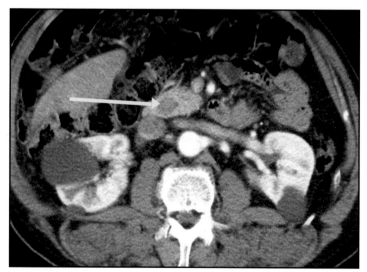

Figure 52-1. Contrast-enhanced axial CT image. (Reprinted with permission from Courtney Moreno, MD, Emory University.)

▶ *What is the diagnosis?*

Vignette 52: Answer

This patient has annular pancreas, which is a rare congenital anomaly resulting from failure of the ventral bud of the pancreas to migrate posteriorly with the duodenum. As a result, a ring of pancreatic tissue encircles the second portion of the duodenum (arrow in Figure 52-1). The classic finding on abdominal X-ray is the "double bubble sign" due to gas in the stomach and also in a dilated duodenal bulb. A pancreatogram can demonstrate an additional ring-like pancreatic duct encircling the second portion of the duodenum, along with a normal main pancreatic duct.

Annular pancreas may be found incidentally. If the anomaly is detected in an asymptomatic patient, then no specific therapy is necessary. On the other hand, this patient with symptoms of duodenal obstruction should undergo surgical bypass of the annulus (with gastrojejunostomy, duodenoduodenostomy, or duodenojejunostomy).

Besides being able to recognize annular pancreas, you should know that these patients have a high prevalence of pancreas divisum. Also, annular pancreas seems to increase the risk of developing an ampullary adenoma (so perform a side-viewing endoscopic examination if a patient with annular pancreas has otherwise unexplained jaundice).

Here's the Point!

Distal duodenal obstruction + Pancreatic tissue encircling duodenum = Annular pancreas

Vignette 53: Panc Ache

A 54-year-old man is seen in clinic for several months of severe, disabling, and constant gnawing epigastric pain radiating to the back. He has consumed a heavy amount of alcohol for the last 30 years. He denies any fevers, chills, or diarrhea. He has lost 5 lb in the last 6 months. He continues to drink a 6 pack of beer daily, and smokes a half pack of cigarettes a day. Vital signs are temperature 98.8°F, blood pressure 130/80 mm Hg, pulse 90 beats/minute, and oxygen saturation 100% on room air. On physical examination, there is mild tenderness to palpation in the epigastrium. Complete blood count, serum chemistry, amylase, and lipase are normal. On CT scan, there are numerous pancreatic parenchymal calcifications. The pancreatic duct is dilated to 7 mm at the body and tail. He refuses any invasive procedures.

▶ *What is the diagnosis?*

▶ *What lifestyle measures and medications can you recommend to ameliorate this patient's abdominal pain?*

Vignette 53: Answer

This patient has chronic pancreatitis. He has a longstanding history of alcohol use and a classic symptom pattern. He has characteristic findings for chronic pancreatitis on CT scan, including pancreatic calcifications and main pancreatic duct dilation. Had this patient undergone endoscopic ultrasound, other features would include an irregular main pancreatic duct with visible side branches, parenchymal lobularity, hyperechoic foci and strands, and hyperechoic margins of the main pancreatic duct.

The 2 major clinical manifestations of chronic pancreatitis are abdominal pain and malabsorption from pancreatic insufficiency. This patient has abdominal pain but no diarrhea, which is not unusual since clinically significant fat and protein deficiencies do not occur until >90% of pancreatic function is lost.

The most important lifestyle measures you should recommend are alcohol and smoking cessation. Alcohol abstinence does not always improve pain but continued alcohol use increases mortality in chronic pancreatitis. Continued tobacco use not only accelerates progression of chronic pancreatitis, but also increases the risk of pancreatic adenocarcinoma. Small meals that are low in fat may provide symptomatic benefit.

Although results from clinical trials show mixed results, some gastroenterologists have used nonenteric coated pancreatic enzyme supplementation for pain relief in chronic pancreatitis. The rationale for the use of pancreatic enzymes for pain relief in chronic pancreatitis is that activated pancreatic enzymes in the duodenum inhibit cholecystokinin (CCK) release. Reduced CCK leads to decreased stimulation of the pancreas. Patients taking an uncoated pancreatic enzyme supplement for chronic pancreatitis pain relief should also take a proton pump inhibitor or an H2 blocker, because gastric acid can inactivate pancreatic enzymes. Nonopioid and opioid analgesics may be options as a last resort for patients with persistent pain despite other therapies, but with the growing opioid epidemic in the United States we need to be extremely careful about starting opioids for long-term use (although it can be hard to refuse opioids in patients with chronic pancreatitis).

This particular patient was not interested in an invasive procedure. If he did wish to consider invasive options, then we could consider offering endoscopy or surgery to help. You should know that an ERCP is most likely to be effective when it is targeted towards treating a stricture or stone proximal to the dilated portion of the main pancreatic duct. However, the endoscopic route seems to be a short-term benefit and may be considered for patients who are not surgical candidates. Surgical decompression with a lateral pancreaticojejunostomy (Puestow procedure) is considered for patients with a dilated main pancreatic duct (usually >6 mm), where it can be durable and very effective, particularly when the pancreas is calcified and hard because the anastomosis is solid and postoperative leaks are uncommon. Surgical resection of the affected portion of the pancreas may be an option for patients with a nondilated main pancreatic duct (ie small duct disease). Prior to any resection, you should counsel patients about the risk of developing endocrine and exocrine dysfunction. In patients with normal pancreatic parenchyma, only about 20% of the pancreas is needed to maintain adequate function. So the majority may be resected if needed for other reasons. However, patients with chronic pancreatitis may not have any normal remaining pancreas, so even a partial pancreatic resection can lead to endocrine and exocrine dysfunction.

Clinical Threshold Alert 1: Clinically significant fat and protein deficiencies do not occur until > 90% of pancreatic function is lost.

Clinical Threshold Alert 2: Main pancreatic duct needs to be greater than 6 mm to derive benefit from surgical decompression in chronic pancreatitis.

Here's the Point!

Alcohol and smoking cessation are critical lifestyle interventions to recommend in chronic pancreatitis.

Vignette 54: Exerting Dominance

A 54-year-old man with a longstanding history of primary sclerosing cholangitis (PSC) undergoes ERCP due to recent fevers and right upper quadrant abdominal pain (below in Figure 54-1). His medical history is significant for ulcerative colitis, which is well-controlled with oral mesalamine. He last underwent a colonoscopy 6 months ago, and at that time no polyps or dysplasia was identified. Vital signs are temperature 98.4°F, pulse 85 beats/minute, blood pressure 110/80 mm Hg, and oxygen saturation 100% on room air. On physical exam, there is scleral icterus without spider angiomas, or shifting dullness or asterixis. Liver tests show total bilirubin 3.4 mg/dL, AST 145 U/L, ALT 160 U/L, and alkaline phosphatase 318 U/L. INR is 1.1, creatinine 0.9.

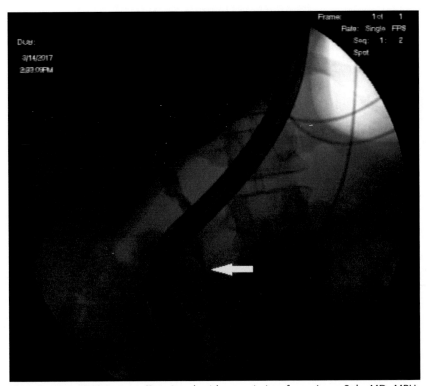

Figure 54-1. ERCP image. (Reprinted with permission from Jung Suh, MD, MPH, Atlanta Gastroenterology Associates.)

▶ *What is the most important finding on the ERCP?*

▶ *What should you do next?*

Vignette 54: Answer

This patient has multiple strictures in the intrahepatic ducts, which is typical for patients with large duct PSC. However, he also has a dominant stricture, (ie a stricture either in the common bile duct, the common hepatic duct, or in the left or right hepatic duct that stands out among the rest). His dominant stricture is in the distal CBD (arrow in Figure 54-1). The major concern here is the possibility that a cholangiocarcinoma could be causing this dominant stricture. PSC patients have a much higher incidence of cholangiocarcinoma than the general population, and PSC patients with dominant strictures have a much higher incidence of cholangiocarcinoma than PSC patients without dominant strictures. In fact, the risk of cholangiocarcinoma is as high as 25% in PSC patients with a dominant stricture.

During the ERCP in a patient with a dominant stricture, it is crucial to obtain tissue samples from the dominant stricture. Modalities of tissue sampling include brushings for cytology and FISH (fluorescence in situ hybridization), regular forceps biopsy under radiographic guidance, or miniforceps biopsy obtained under direct visualization using a cholangioscope. None of the available methods of tissue sampling are terribly sensitive, although they are reasonably specific. CA 19-9 is a serum marker that is often obtained to screen for and diagnose cholangiocarcinoma. Unfortunately, many other benign and malignant gastrointestinal conditions also cause an elevated CA 19-9, which limits this test's specificity.

As an aside, among patients with dominant strictures, you should recognize that *benign* dominant strictures do not routinely worsen cholestasis a large amount. That is, liver tests routinely fluctuate a small extent in patients with PSC, and especially those with cirrhosis. So minor changes in liver tests should not always prompt a referral for endoscopic therapy. In fact, you should be especially cautious about routinely performing ERCP in PSC patients because retained contrast upstream to intrahepatic strictures pose an increased risk of cholangitis or abscess. In fact, PSC is among the few indications for routine pre-ERCP antibiotic prophylaxis (others are cholangitis, malignant hilar obstruction, and biliary complications following liver transplantation).

Sometimes, benign dominant strictures may truly worsen cholestasis or lead to recurrent episodes of cholangitis. In these patients, stricture dilation alone provides similar efficacy with lower complications when compared to dilation and stenting. Therefore, dilation alone is the preferred therapy for treating cholestasis due to a benign dominant stricture.

PSC is the most common cause of sclerosing cholangitis, but other disease processes can cause similar clinical and radiologic findings. Etiologies of secondary sclerosing cholangitis that are important for Board review are summarized in Table 54-1.

Why Might This Be Tested? PSC is a chronic biliary disease that occurs commonly with IBD and therefore is important for the gastroenterologist to understand fully. PSC patients have a significantly elevated risk of cholangiocarcinoma, and you need to know when to do an ERCP or not.

Table 54-1.
ETIOLOGIES OF SECONDARY SCLEROSING CHOLANGITIS

Disease	Pearls
Autoimmune cholangiopathy	Sclerosing cholangitis is the most common extrapancreatic manifestation of type 1 autoimmune pancreatitis. Tissue biopsy demonstrates IgG4-positive plasma cells. The disease usually responds to steroids.
Eosinophilic cholangiopathy	Sclerosing cholangitis with eosinophil infiltrates in the portal triads can occur with drug injury or biliary parasitic infection.
Portal biliopathy	Obstruction of the portal vein due to chronic thrombosis of the portal venous system can cause several venous collaterals to develop to bypass the obstruction. These dilated venous collaterals can cause extrinsic biliary obstruction.
Ischemic cholangitis	The bile duct receives blood supply solely from the hepatic artery. Compromise of blood flow from the hepatic artery to the bile duct can lead to ischemic strictures which can be seen after liver transplantation. The most common setting for ischemic cholangitis is post liver transplantation.
Other	Bile duct stones, trauma, AIDS cholangiopathy, and recurrent pyogenic cholangitis (all discussed in other vignettes).

Here's the Point!

PSC + New dominant stricture → Need to rule out cholangiocarcinoma

Vignette 55: Between a Rock and a Hard Place

A 58-year-old man presents with fever and acute right upper quadrant pain. Initially, he had episodes of right upper quadrant pain after eating a heavy meal, but these episodes typically resolved within 30 minutes. However, now his current symptoms have been persistent for the last 12 hours. His medical history is significant for mitral valve regurgitation requiring placement of a mechanical mitral valve, for which he takes warfarin. On physical examination, he appears uncomfortable. He has scleral icterus. Vital signs are temperature 102.1°F, pulse 115 beats/minute, blood pressure 90/60 mm Hg, respirations 20/minute, and oxygen saturation 98% on room air. Laboratory studies show WBC count 19.4K, hemoglobin 14.1 g/dL, platelets 305, creatinine 2.1 mg/dL, total bilirubin 5.4 mg/dL, alkaline phosphatase 430 U/L, AST 181 U/L, ALT 160 U/L, and INR 3.0. Hydration with normal saline and intravenous antibiotics are initiated. An MRCP is obtained and demonstrates a 12-mm stone in the mid common bile duct. The upstream bile ducts are dilatated to 15 mm.

▶ *What is the next step in management?*

Vignette 55: Answer

The patient has a large bile duct stone and clinical evidence of ascending cholangitis, which is a strong indication to urgently perform an ERCP. Typically, a biliary sphincterotomy is required at the time of ERCP to successfully remove a large bile duct stone. However, this patient is on anticoagulation and has an INR of 3.0, which greatly increases his risk of bleeding after sphincterotomy. On the other hand, reversing his anticoagulation poses an excessively high risk of thrombosis in the setting of a mechanical mitral valve. Therefore, the next step at this time is to perform an ERCP and place a temporary stent without performing sphincterotomy. This maneuver facilitates biliary drainage while minimizing his bleeding risk. Definitive therapy can be attempted at a future date after bridging the patient off warfarin with a short-acting anticoagulant agent like heparin.

This is a perfect time to discuss management of large bile duct stones in the usual instances, when there is normal coagulation. You are probably aware that sphincterotomy followed by stone retrieval with a basket or a balloon is not always successful. A commonly employed approach in this situation is to combine a small biliary sphincterotomy with balloon dilation of the biliary orifice (ie balloon sphincteroplasty). Balloon dilation of the biliary orifice can alter the "cone-shaped" distal tapering to look more like a "cannoli-shaped" distal bile duct, and thus facilitate stone passage. Don't perform balloon sphincteroplasty alone though, because sphincteroplasty without sphincterotomy carries a high risk of pancreatitis. When these standard techniques fail, other options include mechanical lithotripsy (devices that break stones captured in a basket), electrohydraulic lithotripsy (device that is advanced up to the stone under cholangioscopic guidance and delivers shock waves to break up stones), laser lithotripsy, and extracorporeal shock wave lithotripsy. There is no universal consensus as to which of these methods to attempt first after standard techniques (sphincterotomy +/− sphincteroplasty and balloon or basket extraction) fail to retrieve the stone.

Why Might This Be Tested? Ascending cholangitis is one of the few indications for an urgent ERCP. When ascending cholangitis occurs in a patient with a strong indication for anticoagulation, you should know the optimal approach to relieving biliary obstruction while minimizing bleeding risk.

Here's the Point!

Large bile duct stone + Ascending cholangitis + Patient on anticoagulation = Place a stent without performing sphincterotomy during ERCP

Vignette 56: Stricture Picture

A 50-year-old man is seen in clinic 2 months after undergoing liver transplantation for hepatitis C cirrhosis. His immediate post-transplant course was unremarkable. He does not report any specific complaints. His medications include tacrolimus and mycophenolate mofetil. On physical examination, there is scleral icterus. His surgical site appears clean, dry, and intact. He has no tenderness to palpation. Vital signs are temperature 98.6°F, pulse 85 beats/minute, blood pressure 120/80 mm Hg, respirations 12/minute, and oxygen saturation 99% on room air. Routine liver tests obtained immediately prior to his appointment are total bilirubin 4 mg/dL, direct bilirubin 3.5 mg/dL, alkaline phosphatase 643 U/L, AST 180 U/L, ALT 200 U/L, and INR 1.2. A Doppler ultrasound of the liver demonstrates patent vasculature. An ERCP is obtained (Figure 56-1).

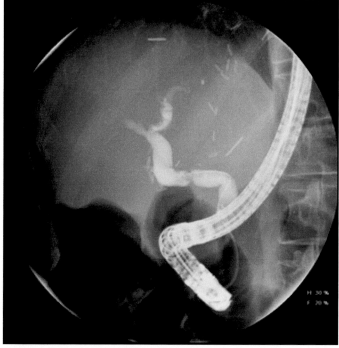

Figure 56-1. ERCP image. (Reprinted with permission from Divyanshoo R. Kohli, MD, Mayo Clinic Arizona.)

▶ *What is the finding on ERCP?*

▶ *What should you recommend next?*

▶ *What other conditions can cause a similar pattern of liver enzyme elevation in this setting?*

Vignette 56: Answer

This patient has a post-transplant stricture at the biliary anastomosis. The clue to recognize on ERCP (or MRCP) is that the area of narrowing is near the surgical clips, at the level of the common hepatic duct (which is the site of the recipient bile duct to donor bile duct anastomosis). Most anastomotic strictures occur within the first 12 months after a liver transplant. Patients with anastomotic strictures are frequently asymptomatic, as was the case with the patient in this vignette. In the early postoperative period, these strictures typically occur because of ischemia or fibrosis from suboptimal surgical technique (eg bile leak, excessive use of electrocautery, inappropriate suture material, or tension at the anastomosis). Small caliber bile ducts or a mismatch in size between the donor and recipient bile ducts also increase the risk of developing an anastomotic stricture.

ERCP with balloon dilation of the stricture and stent placement is usually successful for stricture resolution. This often requires multiple ERCP sessions every 3 months over the course of 1 to 2 years. Placing multiple side-by-side stents across the stricture increases the likelihood of resolving the stricture when compared to repeatedly placing a single stent. Success rates are high with endoscopic therapy, but sometimes the stricture will persist despite multiple ERCP sessions. These patients that do not respond to endoscopic means, typically require surgical intervention, ie a Roux-en-Y hepaticojejunostomy or Roux-en-Y choledochojejunostomy.

Besides anastomotic strictures, other common causes of post-transplant cholestasis are also important to know. Stones, sludge, and cast material can all cause biliary obstruction and can be removed at the time of an ERCP. You should assess for hepatic artery stenosis with a Doppler ultrasound in any liver transplant patient with evidence of cholestasis as well, especially in the early postoperative period. Decreased blood flow to the liver and biliary tree from hepatic artery stenosis can cause liver infarcts and ischemic biliary strictures. The treatment for a patient with hepatic artery stenosis is percutaneous angioplasty or surgical revision—not an ERCP.

You should also know that the hepatitis C virus (HCV) almost universally recurs following liver transplant in those who do not achieve a sustained virologic response to therapy. In about 5% to 10% of patients, HCV reinfection manifests as rapidly progressive cholestatic hepatitis with portal fibrosis leading to graft failure termed fibrosing cholestatic hepatitis (FCH). Patients with FCH traditionally had a very poor prognosis, even with retransplantation. However, direct-acting antiviral agents (DAAs) have drastically improved outcomes in FCH as well. Specific DAA regimens for HCV treatment are ever changing and are continually updated as more data becomes available with newer agents.

Why Might This Be Tested? The biliary tract is the most common site of postoperative complications after liver transplantation, and strictures are the most common biliary complication after liver transplant. Prompt recognition and endoscopic treatment with stricture dilation and stenting can save your patient from requiring another operation, including possible need for retransplantation.

Here's the Point!

**Liver transplant + Cholestasis + Patent hepatic artery on ultrasound =
Suspect an anastomotic biliary stricture**

Vignette 57: The Rolling Stones

A 75-year-old woman presents to the emergency department with 48 hours of constant right upper quadrant pain. She has a history of obesity, hypertension, and type 2 diabetes. She does not smoke or drink alcohol or use any illicit drugs. Medications include aspirin, lisinopril, hydrochlorothiazide, and metformin. On physical examination, she appears uncomfortable, with tenderness in the right upper quadrant. Vital signs are temperature 101.6°F, heart rate 100 beats/minute, blood pressure 110/80 mm Hg, respirations 15/minute, and oxygen saturation 94% on room air. Laboratory studies show WBC count 14.8K, hemoglobin 13 g/dL, platelets 300K, total bilirubin 1 mg/dL, alkaline phosphatase 98 U/L, AST 95 U/L, and ALT 87 U/L. A right upper quadrant ultrasound is obtained and demonstrates several large gallstones in the gallbladder with wall thickening and pericholecystic fluid, all suggestive of acute cholecystitis. She is admitted to the hospital and initiated on intravenous fluids and intravenous antibiotics. Within 24 hours, her symptoms begin to improve. She is discharged home with a plan to perform a cholecystectomy within 2 weeks. However, 10 days later, she presents with episodic diffuse abdominal discomfort, nausea, and vomiting. Laboratory studies are WBC count 11.8K, hemoglobin 12.9 g/dL, platelets 320K, total bilirubin 1 mg/dL, alkaline phosphatase 95 U/L, AST 46 U/L, and ALT 42 U/L. A CT scan of the abdomen is performed showing the following images (Figures 57-1 and 57-2).

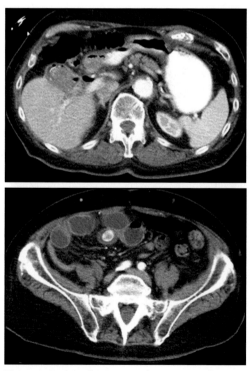

Figures 57-1 and 57-2. Axial contrast enhanced CT images. (Reprinted with permission from Courtney Moreno, MD, Emory University.)

▶ *What's going on here?*

▶ *Why did these symptoms occur?*

Vignette 57: Answer

This patient with acute calculous cholecystitis initially improved with intravenous fluids and antibiotics, but now has recurrent symptoms because of a gallstone ileus. Pericholecystic inflammation can predispose to adhesions, typically between the gallbladder and the duodenum in most of these cases. This can lead to a biliary enteric fistula, which serves as a portal for gallstones to migrate right into the small intestine ("The Rolling Stones"). As the stone migrates distally, it can get impacted in the small intestine and cause symptoms of bowel obstruction. Symptoms improve when the gallstone gets disimpacted and tumbles distally but recurs when the stone lodges in the more distal small bowel. Most stones that cause gallstone ileus are >2 cm in size, and the most common site of impaction is the ileum, since it's the narrowest part of the small intestine. The condition seems to occur most frequently in elderly women.

This patient has several characteristic imaging findings of gallstone ileus. On the first image above, air is seen in the gallbladder wall with thickening of the gallbladder reflecting inflammation. On the second image, a large gallstone in the small bowel is seen with upstream dilated small bowel loops. Did you catch that? Sometimes in these cases, you can see air in the biliary tree (pneumobilia) from the cholecystoenteric fistula. You should know that pneumobilia also occurs after a biliary sphincterotomy. In the setting of a biliary sphincterotomy, pneumobilia is actually a good thing since it confirms that the sphincterotomy is patent. By the way, the triad of dilated small bowel loops, pneumobilia, and a radiopaque density in the small bowel is called "Rigler's Triad." This triad can sometimes be captured on a plain abdominal X-ray if the gallstone happens to be radiopaque. However, these days we seem to jump straight to a CT scan for diagnosis.

Once you have diagnosed a patient as having gallstone ileus, the next step is to call your surgeon to perform an enterolithotomy. If the patient is a reasonable operative candidate, the surgeon should perform a cholecystectomy and fistula division as well to reduce the risk of recurrent gallstone ileus.

Besides the small intestine, gallstones can lodge in other areas of the gastrointestinal tract and cause various interesting (and uncomfortable!) syndromes. Bouveret syndrome occurs when a large gallstone causes gastric outlet obstruction by impaction of the gallstone at the pylorus through a cholecystogastric fistula or impaction at the duodenum creating proximal gastric outlet obstruction. Mirizzi's syndrome is obstructive jaundice that occurs when a large gallstone becomes impacted in the gallbladder infundibulum or cystic duct and compresses the extrahepatic bile duct (Figure 57-3).

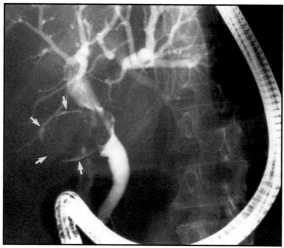

Figure 57-3. Mirizzi's syndrome with contrast outlining a large stone (arrows) impacted in the cystic duct and compressing the bile duct. (Reprinted with permission from Anthony J. DiMarino Jr, MD and Stanley B. Benjamin, MD.)

Here's the Point! 1

Pneumobilia + Small bowel obstruction + Large gallstone in GI tract = Gallstone ileus

Here's the Point! 2

Epigastric pain + Succussion splash + Large gallstone near pylorus= Bouveret syndrome

Here's the Point! 3

Obstructive jaundice + Gallstone in GB neck or cystic duct compressing common hepatic duct = Mirizzi's syndrome

Here's the Point! 4

Dilated small bowel loops + Pneumobilia + Radiopaque density in small bowel = Rigler's Triad

Vignette 58: A Rocky Pregnancy

A 32-year-old woman presents with 3 hours of right upper quadrant pain. Symptoms began after consuming a cheeseburger and french fries. She has experienced similar episodes over the last month, but her prior symptoms typically resolved within 30 minutes. She is currently in her first trimester of pregnancy. On physical examination, she appears uncomfortable. There is tenderness to palpation of the right upper quadrant without rebound or guarding. Vital signs are temperature 98.7°F, heart rate 95 beats/minute, blood pressure 110/80 mm Hg, respirations 15/minute, and oxygen saturation 96% on room air. Her body mass index is 40. Laboratory studies are WBC count 10.3K, hemoglobin 13 g/dL, platelets 300K, total bilirubin 2.9 mg/dL, alkaline phosphatase 285 U/L, AST 117 U/L, and ALT 121 U/L. A right upper quadrant ultrasound is obtained and demonstrates several large gallstones. The common bile duct is dilated to 10 mm, but no common bile duct stones are visualized.

▶ *What's going on here?*

▶ *What test can you perform to confirm the diagnosis?*

Vignette 58: Answer

This patient has gallstones, and likely also has a stone in her common bile duct. Pregnancy increases the risk of gallstone formation by the increased hormonal levels. Cholesterol becomes supersaturated by estrogen increasing cholesterol secretion and by progesterone decreasing bile acid secretion. Moreover, progesterone also slows gallbladder emptying, resulting in gallbladder stasis. Obesity is also a major risk factor for gallstone formation. Therefore, it is not surprising that this woman has gallstones.

Transabdominal ultrasound is not terribly sensitive at detecting bile duct stones, so you cannot rule out choledocholithiasis based solely on the negative right upper quadrant ultrasound. A CT scan would expose the fetus to ionizing radiation, and is therefore avoided during pregnancy. MRI is generally not recommended in the first trimester because of a theoretical risk of teratogenicity. If this patient were in the second or third trimester, then a noncontrast MRI would have been an acceptable imaging modality.

EUS is highly sensitive and specific at detecting bile duct stones, and does not expose the patient to ionizing radiation. If EUS demonstrates a stone in the common bile duct, then an ERCP is safe to perform during pregnancy and is recommended to reduce the risk of cholangitis and pancreatitis. The endoscopist can reduce fetal radiation exposure by minimizing fluoroscopy time, avoiding fluoroscopic image magnification, and avoiding spot films. Placing a lead apron or shield below the patient is also recommended, although this strategy does not prevent fetal exposure to internally scattered radiation (remember that the radiation source is below the patient so you should also place the shield below the patient).

As of 2015, the Food and Drug Administration no longer assigns pregnancy risk categories (A, B, C, D, X) to drugs in the United States. Instead, they want providers to make individualized decisions about risks and benefits during pregnancy or postpartum based upon available human and animal studies and potential or known adverse reactions. It is then up to the provider to figure out if the dose should be reduced, or if the medication should be given at all. With that in mind, meperidine or propofol tend to work pretty well for ERCP during pregnancy. Of note, benzodiazepines should generally be avoided in pregnancy, especially in the first trimester.

Following ERCP, this patient should undergo a cholecystectomy. Supportive care is a reasonable strategy in a pregnant woman with a single episode of biliary colic but would not be appropriate for this woman with recurrent episodes of biliary colic complicated by choledocholithiasis. Laparoscopic cholecystectomy should be performed at any stage of pregnancy in patients with a strong indication for the operation (although the surgery may be more technically challenging in the late third trimester). Pregnancy alone does not increase postoperative morbidity after a cholecystectomy, and a laparoscopic approach does not worsen fetal outcomes. See the first *Acing* book for more information on managing gallstones in pregnancy.

Why Might This Be Tested? Three reasons: Gallstone disease is common, pregnancy increases the risk of this common condition, and the management of GI diseases during pregnancy is very important for Board review.

Here's the Point!

Pregnancy + Bile duct stones = EUS is a safe, sensitive, and specific diagnostic test; ERCP and cholecystectomy can be performed in any trimester

Vignettes 59-62: Good Gally!

We all learned to recognize and manage gallstone-related cholecystitis in medical school. A patient with a sudden cessation of inspiration due to pain with palpation under the right costal margin (ie "Murphy's sign") and ultrasound findings of gallbladder wall thickening and pericholecystic fluid should not pose much of a diagnostic dilemma. On the other hand, nongallstone related cholecystitis and swelling are more challenging to recognize, but their consequences can be just as deleterious. Good "gally" you will need to know what to do! For each of the vignettes below, identify the most likely diagnosis and subsequent management.

59.   A 78-year-old man is admitted to the intensive care unit for hypotension following an abdominal aortic aneurysm repair. Three days later, he develops fever, leukocytosis, and right upper quadrant pain. Right upper quadrant ultrasound demonstrates gallbladder wall thickening and a round pericholecystic fluid collection, but no gallstones.

60.   An 80-year-old man with a history of end stage renal disease, congestive heart failure, and diabetes mellitus develops pneumonia requiring intubation and admission to the intensive care unit. He is extubated after 48 hours and subsequently develops right upper quadrant pain, fever, leukocytosis, and hypotension requiring pressor support. On physical examination, there is right upper quadrant crepitus. Total bilirubin is 2.8 mg/dL, and unconjugated bilirubin is 2.2 mg/dL.

61.   A 48-year-old Asian woman is admitted with acute onset of fever, right upper quadrant pain, and leukocytosis. A right upper quadrant ultrasound reveals gallstones, a 9-mm gallbladder wall, and round hypoechoic nodules within the gallbladder wall.

62.   A 50-year-old woman presents to the emergency department with hematuria and right flank pain. A noncontrast abdominal CT does not show evidence of the suspected nephrolithiasis. However, one of the axial images reveals the finding shown below in Figure 62-1.

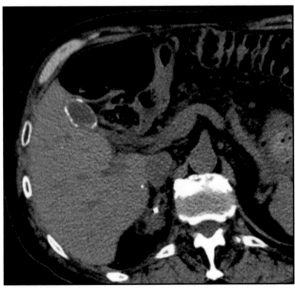

Figure 62-1. Axial noncontrast CT scan. (Reprinted with permission from Courtney Moreno, MD, Emory University.)

Vignettes 59-62: Answers

59. This is acalculous cholecystitis. Critical illness predisposes to gallbladder stasis and ischemia, which can result in gallbladder wall inflammation. Because critically ill patients are often unable to provide history, unexplained fever and leukocytosis are often the only signs of acalculous cholecystitis. In addition, since the presentation can be insidious, these patients can often develop secondary infection, gallbladder gangrene, and subsequent gallbladder perforation. As a result, acalculous cholecystitis carries a very high mortality rate. Once you diagnose a patient with acalculous cholecystitis, you should obtain blood cultures to help guide antibiotic therapy and promptly initiate broad-spectrum antibiotics. You should also obtain an abdominal X-ray to assess for gallbladder perforation. Patients in the intensive care unit with acalculous cholecystitis are often too ill to undergo a cholecystectomy. If surgery is contraindicated and there is no perforation, you should recommend urgent placement of a cholecystostomy tube.

Here's the Point!

Critically ill patient + Fever, leukocytosis + Gallbladder wall thickening, pericholecystic fluid but no gallstones = Acalculous cholecystitis; start antibiotics and place cholecystostomy tube

60. This patient has emphysematous cholecystitis, which occurs due to secondary infection of the gallbladder with gas-forming organisms. The most common organisms associated with emphysematous cholecystitis are *Clostridium*, *Escherichia coli*, and *Klebsiella* species. Emphysematous cholecystitis disproportionately affects older men with diabetes, like the patient in this vignette. Right upper quadrant crepitus is sometimes appreciated on examination, and is an important diagnostic clue. *Clostridium* species can cause hemolysis, which is likely why this patient has an unconjugated hyperbilirubinemia. The characteristic finding on imaging is air within the gallbladder wall (arrow in Figure 60-1). Like acalculous cholecystitis, patients with emphysematous cholecystitis have a very high risk of developing gallbladder gangrene and perforation, so the mortality associated with this condition is high. Management is similar to acalculous cholecystitis.

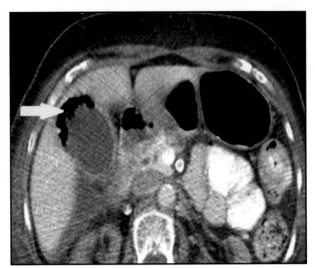

Figure 60-1. Emphysematous cholecystitis. (Reprinted with permission from Courtney Moreno, MD, Emory University.)

Here's the Point!

Elderly + Right upper quadrant pain with Right upper quadrant crepitus = Emphysematous cholecystitis

61.   This patient has xanthogranulomatous cholecystitis. This rare inflammatory condition of the gallbladder is more common among Asians, and occurs more frequently in women. Almost all patients with xanthogranulomatous cholecystitis have gallstones, which may be involved in gallbladder mucosal ulceration or rupture of the gallbladder wall pseudodiverticula (called Rokitansky-Aschoff sinuses). Bile can extravasate into the gallbladder, inciting an inflammatory interstitial reaction. Inflammatory cells phagocytose bile, cholesterol, and phospholipids, leading to the formation of yellow nodules and plaques (xanthomas). On ultrasound, xanthomas appear as hypoechoic nodules or bands. Although extensive inflammation can mimic gallbladder carcinoma, xanthogranulomatous cholecystitis is not a malignant condition. The inflammatory process can be quite severe and extend to adjacent structures, so a cholecystectomy is mandatory. Due to the dense fibrous adhesions in the gallbladder serosa, an open cholecystectomy is usually needed rather than the laparoscopic approach. *Clinical Threshold Alert:* Normal gallbladder wall thickness is < 3 mm.

Here's the Point!

Asian woman + Cholecystitis + Hypoechoic nodules in gallbladder wall = Xanthogranulomatous cholecystitis

62. The CT scan demonstrates intramural calcification of the gallbladder wall. This finding is also termed "porcelain gallbladder," because gross examination would reveal a brittle gallbladder with a bluish hue. The pathogenesis is not entirely clear, but may be related to chronic gallbladder inflammation due to gallstones. Most patients with porcelain gallbladder are asymptomatic, although some patients may have chronic right upper quadrant pain. Interestingly, incomplete gallbladder wall calcification (as shown in Figure 62-1) increases the risk of gallbladder cancer even more than patients with complete mural calcification. Because of this increased gallbladder cancer risk, all patients with porcelain gallbladder should be considered for elective cholecystectomy.

Here's the Point!

Gallbladder wall calcification = Porcelain gallbladder = Increased gallbladder cancer risk

Vignettes 63-65: Iatrogenica Imperfecta

Laparoscopic cholecystectomy is a very safe procedure with a serious complication rate less than 3%. However, since hundreds of thousands of laparoscopic cholecystectomies are performed annually in the United States, you are likely to encounter many patients with a complication related to this surgery. Some of these complications can be managed endoscopically, while others require surgery or another management approach. For each of the following vignettes, identify the most likely cholecystectomy-related complication and its management.

63.   A 35-year-old woman undergoes a laparoscopic cholecystectomy for symptomatic choleli-thiasis. The procedure is uneventful, and she is discharged home 6 hours after the surgery. Two days later, she presents with worsening right upper quadrant pain. On examination, she appears uncomfortable. There is tenderness to palpation in the right upper quadrant. A right upper quadrant ultrasound is obtained and demonstrates a 5-cm fluid collection in the gallbladder fossa. An ERCP is performed (Figure 63-1). Name the diagnosis and its management.

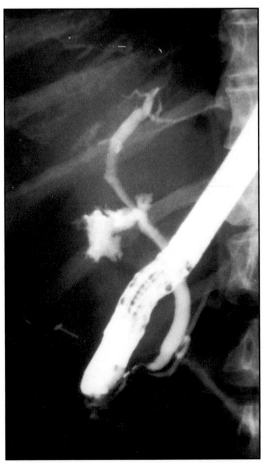

Figure 63-1. ERCP image. (Reprinted with permission from Anthony J. DiMarino Jr, MD and Stanley B. Benjamin, MD.)

64. Three weeks after undergoing a laparoscopic cholecystectomy for biliary dyskinesia, a 45-year-old man is admitted with right upper quadrant pain. Vital signs show a temperature 98.6°F, blood pressure 100/60 mm Hg, heart rate 105 beats/minute, respirations 20/minute, and oxygen saturation 96% on room air. On physical exam, he appears uncomfortable with tenderness to palpation in the right upper quadrant but no rebound tenderness or guarding. There is scleral icterus. Liver tests reveal total bilirubin 3.2 mg/dL, alkaline phosphatase 301 U/L, AST 89 U/L, and ALT 90 U/L. INR is 1.0. An ERCP is performed (Figure 64-1). Name the diagnosis and its management.

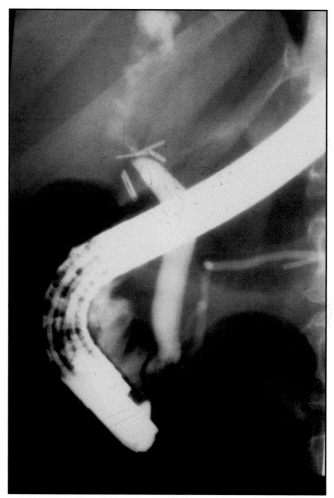

Figure 64-1. ERCP image. (Reprinted with permission from Anthony J. DiMarino Jr, MD and Stanley B. Benjamin, MD.)

65.   Two years after undergoing a cholecystectomy for biliary dyskinesia, a 38-year-old woman begins to experience episodes of severe right upper quadrant pain lasting 30 to 60 minutes. In between episodes she is completely asymptomatic. Episodes occur once or twice a month, but have been increasing in frequency. Laboratory studies obtained in the emergency department during one of her symptomatic episodes are significant for WBC count 5K, total bilirubin 2.0 mg/dL, alkaline phosphatase 200 U/L, AST 200 U/L, and ALT 250 U/L. An MRI obtained during the symptomatic episode demonstrated a 15-mm common bile duct without any stones. When she is asymptomatic, her liver tests are normal and common bile duct diameter is 6 mm.

Vignettes 63-65: Answers

63.   The fluid collection is a biloma from a bile leak at the cystic duct stump. Small fluid collections in the gallbladder bed are very common after cholecystectomy. These small collections typically result from ducts in the gallbladder bed and are usually clinically insignificant. In contrast, large symptomatic bilomas most commonly result from leakage at the cystic duct remnant. Common causes of bile leak from the cystic duct stump include surgical clip displacement or misplacement, and necrosis or tearing of the duct remnant proximal to the clip. The next step is to perform an ERCP to confirm the diagnosis and localize the site of the bile duct leak. Once ERCP confirms a bile duct leak, the patient should have a biliary stent placed across the major papilla for 4 to 6 weeks. The goal of stent placement is to eliminate the transpapillary pressure gradient, so bile flows preferentially through the stent and out of the ampulla rather than the site of the leak (ie bile follows the path of least resistance). Another reasonable alternative is to perform a biliary sphincterotomy to eliminate the transpapillary gradient. Once the leak has resolved, the biloma often reabsorbs rapidly. In some patients with significantly symptomatic bilomas, a percutaneous drain may be necessary.

Here's the Point!

Recent cholecystectomy + Right upper quadrant pain + Right upper quadrant fluid collection = Biloma from a bile duct leak

64.   The cholangiogram demonstrates the common bile duct transected by a surgical clip. This complication usually occurs when the bile duct is mistakenly identified as the cystic duct. Complete transection of the bile duct can present with jaundice even many weeks after the surgery. Longstanding obstruction to bile flow can lead to secondary cirrhosis if repair is not accomplished in a timely manner. The next step is to obtain a percutaneous transhepatic cholangiogram. This procedure should demonstrate dilatated intrahepatic bile ducts proximal to the transection, define the length of the stricture, and allow for decompression of the bile ducts to reduce the risk of cholangitis. Percutaneous decompression is only a temporary solution however. Definitive therapy usually requires surgical hepaticojejunostomy.

Here's the Point!

Jaundice after cholecystectomy + No proximal bile duct opacification on ERCP + Surgical clip in vicinity of bile duct = Bile duct transection

65. Just as disordered relaxation of the pancreatic sphincter of Oddi (SO) could predispose to pancreatitis, disordered relaxation of the biliary SO could lead to symptoms of biliary colic and biliary obstruction even in the absence of a gallbladder or bile duct stones. This patient with recurrent biliary colic after cholecystectomy, dilated bile duct (> 10 mm) and elevated transaminases during episodes without any stones or sludge has biliary SO stenosis (previously termed type 1 biliary SOD). A biliary sphincterotomy without further testing is recommended for this condition. Patients with biliary colic and either a dilated common bile duct or elevated transaminases during episodes may have functional biliary SOD (previously termed type 2 SOD). In these patients, Rome IV guidelines suggest biliary manometry as a reasonable diagnostic test. Biliary manometry is considered abnormal if SO pressure is sustainably greater than 40 mm Hg in both leads across multiple stations. If manometry is abnormal, then biliary sphincterotomy may allow for symptom improvement. Also recall that patients with suspected SOD should receive a pancreatic stent and periprocedural rectal NSAIDs since they have a high risk of developing post-ERCP pancreatitis.

As is the case with pancreatic SOD, Rome IV guidelines do not consider type 3 SOD as a separate diagnostic entity anymore. ERCP is more likely to hurt these patients than to provide any symptomatic benefit. So, don't perform ERCP in patients with recurrent biliary colic but without elevated transaminases or bile duct dilation during the colic episodes.

This patient originally underwent a cholecystectomy for biliary dyskinesia, which is a functional gallbladder disorder, and is a diagnosis of exclusion. To consider the diagnosis of biliary dyskinesia, a patient with biliary type pain must have testing to exclude other causes of pain such as gallstones, sludge, and other intrinsic panc-bil disease or peptic ulcer disease. You can directly test for this gallbladder motility disorder using a hepatobiliary (HIDA) scan. Following an overnight fast, a radiolabeled tracer is injected intravenously and is then excreted in bile. When radioactivity is maximal from the gallbladder and minimal from the liver, cholecystokinin is administered to stimulate the gallbladder to contract, and gallbladder ejection fraction is measured. Gallbladder ejection fraction <40% can help to predict that the patient's symptoms may potentially improve with a cholecystectomy. However, surgery should be considered a last resort. *Clinical Threshold Alert:* HIDA scan is considered suggestive of biliary dyskinesia when biliary pain coincides with gallbladder ejection fraction <40%.

Here's the Point!

Episodes of right upper quadrant pain after cholecystectomy + Bile duct dilation and elevated transaminases during symptomatic episodes + Normalization of liver enzymes and bile duct dilation between episodes = Biliary sphincter of Oddi stenosis (previously termed type 1 SOD)

Vignette 66: Clogged Drain

A 42-year-old man presents with several weeks of right upper quadrant pain and watery diarrhea. The pain is dull and constant but worsens with meals. The diarrhea is large volume, unrelated to meals, and often awakens him. He has a history of human immunodeficiency virus (HIV) infection. He does not take any medications. Vital signs are temperature 98.9°F, blood pressure 101/75 mm Hg, heart rate 98 beats/minute, and oxygen saturation 100% on room air. On physical exam, there is no scleral icterus and mild discomfort to palpation in the right upper quadrant without overt tenderness, rebound, or guarding. Laboratory studies are significant for WBC count 1.5K, CD4 count 50/mm^3, hemoglobin 10.1 g/dL, total bilirubin 1.7 mg/dL, alkaline phosphatase 810 U/L, AST 127 U/L, and ALT 150 U/L. An MRCP demonstrates multiple intrahepatic biliary strictures and extrahepatic bile duct dilation with smooth distal tapering towards the ampulla.

▶ *What's going on here?*

▶ *How should you treat this patient?*

Vignette 66: Answer

This patient has AIDS cholangiopathy (ERCP image shown below in Figure 66-1), which occurs due to infection-related strictures in the biliary tract. AIDS cholangiopathy typically occurs when a patient's CD4 count falls below 100/mm^3. The organism most frequently implicated is *Cryptosporidium parvum*, although cytomegalovirus (CMV), *Cyclospora*, and *Microsporidium* have also been identified. The intrahepatic strictures appear similar on cholangiography to primary sclerosing cholangitis (PSC). Unlike PSC, however, most patients with AIDS cholangiopathy also have papillary stenosis, which is why this patient has a dilated extrahepatic duct with smooth distal tapering towards the ampulla. The most common symptoms are abdominal pain (due to the papillary stenosis) and diarrhea (from parasitic infection of the GI tract).

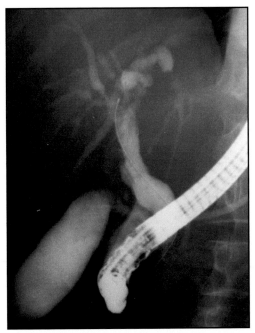

Figure 66-1. HIV/AIDS cholangiopathy. (Reprinted with permission from Anthony J. DiMarino Jr, MD and Stanley B. Benjamin, MD.)

Survival in AIDS cholangiopathy is related primarily to the natural history of AIDS, so you should recommend highly active antiretroviral therapy (HAART). Immune reconstitution with HAART should reduce mortality, rid the body of *Cryptosporidium* and help resolve the patient's diarrhea. However, we don't know if HAART improves abdominal pain or biliary strictures in AIDS cholangiopathy. The primary treatment for abdominal pain in AIDS cholangiopathy with papillary stenosis is to perform an ERCP with biliary sphincterotomy. Dilation and stenting of dominant strictures may improve jaundice, but are not typically effective in patients with multiple intrahepatic strictures.

AIDS cholangiopathy was quite common in the era before HAART became widely available, but its incidence has decreased markedly since that time. Nowadays, abnormal liver tests and cholestasis in patients with HIV/AIDS are far more commonly due to medications than cholangiopathy. For example, trimethoprim-sulfamethoxazole, which is routinely administered to HIV infected patients when their CD4 counts falls below 200/mm^3, can cause an idiosyncratic cholestasis within 2 to 12 weeks of initiation. Also, the antiretrovirals atazanavir and indinavir inhibit UDP glucuronyl transferase, the enzyme that is responsible for conjugation of bilirubin. These antiretroviral agents can cause jaundice from unconjugated hyperbilirubinemia. With AIDS cholangiopathy, there is usually disproportionate elevation in alkaline phosphatase compared with bilirubin, and jaundice is uncommon. However, when jaundice does occur in AIDS cholangiopathy, it is usually due to conjugated hyperbilirubinemia.

Why Might This Be Tested? Not all patients with HIV take HAART and therefore, profound immunosuppression still occurs. A biliary sphincterotomy can lead to significant symptom improvement in patients with AIDS cholangiopathy and papillary stenosis, so you need to consider this etiology in your differential diagnosis.

Here's the Point!

AIDS + CD4 count < 100/mm^3 + Biliary strictures + Papillary stenosis = AIDS cholangiopathy

Vignette 67-69: ERCP Gone Bad

Acute pancreatitis is the most common severe complication of ERCP; its prevention and management rightfully receives a lot of attention. Nonetheless, pancreatitis is certainly not the only adverse event that can occur after an ERCP. For each of the following vignettes, identify the most likely ERCP-related complication and its management.

67.   A 45-year-old woman with episodes of right upper quadrant discomfort is found to have cholelithiasis, including a large stone in the distal bile duct. She undergoes ERCP. Biliary cannulation is challenging and requires a precut papillotomy. After the bile duct is cannulated, a large biliary sphincterotomy is performed, and the stone is successfully removed with a balloon. Following the procedure, the patient reports right upper quadrant pain and back pain. On examination, there is mild tenderness in the right upper quadrant. Vital signs are temperature 36.9°F, blood pressure 130/80 mm Hg, heart rate 88 beats/minute, and oxygen saturation 98% on room air. WBC count and serum lipase are normal. An abdominal MRI is obtained (Figure 67-1).

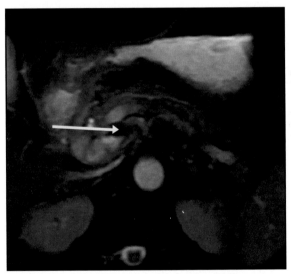

Figure 67-1. T2 weighted MRI image after ERCP.

68. A 50-year-old man with choledocholithiasis undergoes an ERCP. The duodenoscope is passed with ease into the second portion of the duodenum, but multiple attempts to reduce the scope to the "short" position are unsuccessful. The bile duct is easily cannulated in the long position and the stone is removed after a medium sized biliary sphincterotomy and balloon sweep are performed. Immediately after the procedure, the patient reports abdominal pain. Vital signs are temperature 98.4°F, blood pressure 106/67 mm Hg, heart rate 108 beats/minute, and oxygen saturation is 100% on 2 L oxygen. On exam, there is diffuse abdominal tenderness. Serum lipase is normal. A contrast CT scan is immediately obtained (Figure 68-1).

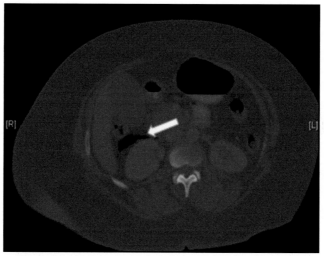

Figure 68-1. Axial contrast enhanced CT scan. (Reprinted with permission from Joel Camilo, MD, Atlanta Gastroenterology Associates.)

69. A 75-year-old man undergoes a second ERCP with monitored anesthesia care to remove a large common bile duct stone using air (not carbon dioxide) insufflation. He had previously undergone ERCP with sphincterotomy and balloon dilation of the biliary orifice followed by unsuccessful attempts using a balloon and an extraction basket. A plastic biliary stent was placed at the time. During this ERCP, the biliary stent is removed and the biliary sphincterotomy is extended. Then, a cholangioscopy with electrohydraulic lithotripsy is performed. Before the remaining stone fragments can be retrieved, his oxygen saturation abruptly drops to 70% on 4 L supplemental oxygen. His heart rate increases to 160 beats/minute, and the rhythm on the monitor indicates a sinus tachycardia. Blood pressure suddenly drops to 70/30 mm Hg. He is observed to have cyanosis of the head, neck, and trunk. There is no free air visible under the diaphragm on fluoroscopy.

Vignette 67-69: Answers

67. The patient has a retroperitoneal perforation, as evidenced by air in the retroperitoneal space (arrow in Figure 67-1). The most commonly recognized risk factors for this complication are precut papillotomy and large biliary sphincterotomy, because the endoscopist can inadvertently extend the cut beyond the major papilla and into the duodenal wall. Another cause of retroperitoneal air is duct perforation, which usually occurs due to forceful advancement of the guidewire. Absence of retroperitoneal air on X-ray does not rule out a retroperitoneal perforation. So, if there is a high index of suspicion with a negative plain film, then you should obtain a CT scan with contrast. This patient was stable and got an MRI and accordingly was admitted for observation, intravenous fluids, and antibiotics. Although surgical consultation is recommended, most of these perforations seal with conservative management alone. However, you should know that a small amount of retroperitoneal air can be seen on a quarter of CT scans immediately after ERCP. In asymptomatic patients, retroperitoneal air is usually not clinically significant, so no specific intervention is necessary.

Here's the Point!

Large biliary sphincterotomy or precut papillotomy + Post-ERCP abdominal pain + Normal serum lipase = Think of retroperitoneal perforation (often responds to conservative management)

68. This patient has free air noted on the CT scan due to a lateral wall perforation (arrow in Figure 68-1). These perforations occur distant to the ampulla, and are usually the result of trauma by the endoscope itself. Postsurgical anatomy (eg Billroth II anatomy) or strictures are the most common risk factors for this uncommon complication. When the duodenoscope is initially advanced to the second portion of the duodenum, the scope typically makes a loop in the stomach. This position is termed the "long" position. Before attempting cannulation, most endoscopists will attempt to reduce the loop in the stomach by withdrawing the scope to the "short" position. Pressure exerted on the lateral duodenal wall during this "shortening" maneuver can also rarely predispose to a lateral duodenal wall perforation. Unlike retroperitoneal perforations, a lateral duodenal wall perforation is unlikely to respond to conservative management. Here, the endoscope was reinserted and demonstrated the perforation with omentum visible (arrow in Figure 68-2). This defect was successfully closed with clips (Figure 68-3).

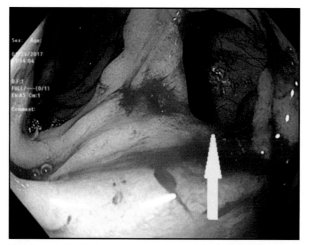

Figure 68-2. Endoscopy revealed perforation of the lateral wall (arrow), opposite the ampulla. (Reprinted with permission from Joel Camilo, MD, Atlanta Gastroenterology Associates.)

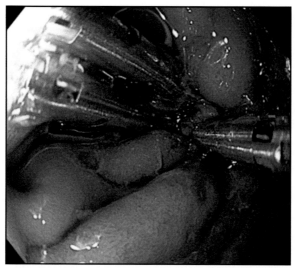

Figure 68-3. Endoscopic clip used for closure. (Reprinted with permission from Joel Camilo, MD, Atlanta Gastroenterology Associates.)

A contrast upper GI series the next day confirmed there was a successful closure with no leak of contrast and the patient did well. However, if the patient is hemodynamically unstable or if endoscopic closure is unable to be performed, then emergent surgery is the next step for a lateral wall perforation. Since we are discussing free air under the diaphragm, you should know that the amount of free air under the diaphragm does not necessarily correlate with the severity of injury. However, a large amount of free air can compress the inferior vena cava which can impair venous return resulting in profound and abrupt hypotension. If your patient acutely develops a tense abdomen and profound hypotension during endoscopy, you should first perform emergent abdominal decompression (eg insert a percutaneous needle or angiocatheter into the abdominal wall) to prevent circulatory collapse.

Here's the Point!

Billroth II anatomy + Post-ERCP abdominal pain + Normal lipase + Free air under the diaphragm = Lateral wall perforation (usually requires emergency surgery)

69.   You should suspect an air embolism in any patient with acute cardiovascular or neurologic collapse during ERCP, particularly if there is no evidence of a free wall perforation. Previous biliary interventions, cholangioscopy, and use of air rather than carbon dioxide for insufflation are all risk factors for this complication. Sphincterotomy and air insufflation can cause air to enter venous radicles close to the papilla and enter the portal venous system. Air insufflated directly into the bile duct can cause air to directly enter the hepatic veins during cholangioscopy. Air in the portal vein or hepatic veins can pass sequentially into the inferior vena cava, the right ventricle, and the pulmonary circulation. The result is a venous air embolism. In patients with a patent foramen ovale, air can enter the arterial system and travel to the cerebral circulation (arterial air embolism). Air embolism during ERCP is rare, but prompt recognition is key because of the high mortality associated with this tragic complication. An emergent bedside echocardiogram is a valuable diagnostic tool, since this test may demonstrate air in the right ventricle. Management is cardiopulmonary resuscitation. If air is seen in the right ventricle on echocardiogram, you or preferably a member of the emergency team could consider aspirating the air via a central venous line. Placing the head down (ie Trendelenburg position) is also generally advocated.

Here's the Point!

Acute cardiovascular or neurologic collapse during ERCP + No free air on fluoroscopy = Suspect air embolism. Put in Trendelenburg and call for help!

Vignette 70: Pancreatic Pebbles

A 48-year-old man with chronic abdominal pain due to chronic pancreatitis is on methadone maintenance. He has been doing a lot of reading about the risks of narcotic dependence and side effects and wishes to avoid taking narcotics. He has been able to keep his job and has also maintained his weight but his abdominal pain is persistent despite previous endoscopic therapy for pancreatic duct stones. His bowel habits are regular and he reports no jaundice or pruritis. He has no history of gallstones or alcohol use. On examination, he appears well nourished and is in no distress. His abdomen is soft and mildly tender diffusely without distention. Laboratory tests show the following: Triglycerides 110 mg/dL, IgG4 58 mg/dL, total bilirubin 1.0, albumin 3.9, ALT 29, lipase 62, WBC 6.1, hemoglobin 14.1, and platelets 195. A CT scan is performed, shown below in Figure 70-1.

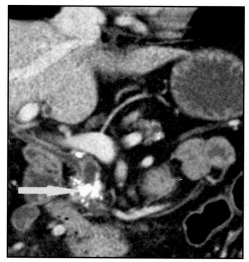

Figure 70-1. Coronal CT image. (Reprinted with permission from Courtney Moreno, MD, Emory University.)

▶ *What should you recommend as the best long-term treatment for his pain?*

Vignette 70: Answer

This patient's pain is due to obstructive chronic pancreatitis with a CT showing a large stone (arrow in Figure 70-1) with a dilated main pancreatic duct. The knee-jerk reaction might be to perform a therapeutic ERCP. However, the best long-term option is surgical decompression of the pancreatic duct, which is typically accomplished with a lateral pancreaticojejunostomy, also known as Puestow procedure (see Vignette 53 for more). Relieving the elevated pressure in the duct is the key for pain reduction. Although there may be short-term gain with endoscopic therapy which could include pancreatic sphincterotomy, dilation of strictures, pancreatic duct stone removal with or without lithotripsy and stent placement, endoscopic therapy rarely provides long term relief and the vast majority of endoscopically treated patients will eventually require surgery. Thus, the most durable form of pain relief in obstructive chronic pancreatitis is surgical therapy. Moreover, a cost utility analysis found that surgical therapy was more cost-effective than endoscopic therapy. In fact, surgical treatment rarely requires an additional drainage procedure, which contrasts with endoscopic therapy. Surgical therapy is also more effective in pain reduction over the long haul compared with celiac plexus neurolysis, pancreatic enzymes, and other pain modulating and dietary strategies. So, the best plan would be to cut to the chase and just go under the knife. That's right: Put that scope down and send your patient to an experienced surgeon.

Why Might This Be Tested? This is a perfect example in a real-world scenario where you have to provide the best plan that requires thinking outside of the endoscopy room. You must know when to hand over a case to your surgical colleagues.

Here's the Point!

Surgical therapy is the best modality for long-term pain relief in obstructive chronic pancreatitis.

Vignette 71: Mahogany Mess

A 54-year-old man with a history of alcoholism has been admitted to the intensive care unit with another bout of severe acute pancreatitis. Upon admission, a CT scan with intravenous contrast was performed and is shown below in Figure 71-1.

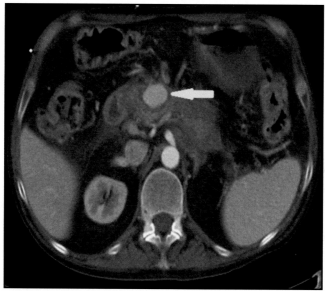

Figure 71-1. Axial contrast enhanced CT image. (Reprinted with permission from Courtney Moreno, MD, Emory University.)

He suddenly develops hypotension and a large volume of mahogany stools in the ICU. Aggressive resuscitation ensues immediately and esophagogastroduodenoscopy is performed. The EGD is notable for blood in the second portion of the duodenum without any mucosal abnormalities. That is, there are no varices or ulcers or arteriovenous malformations found.

▶ *What is the diagnosis?*

Vignette 71: Answer

This is hemosuccus pancreaticus, a rare cause of upper gastrointestinal tract hemorrhage. This has to be the best disease name in gastroenterology. Not based on outcome, but it just sounds so cool. This patient has had rapid bleeding from destruction of the arterial wall of a pseudoaneurysm with blood pouring into the pancreatic duct. Subsequently, this blood then passes through ampulla of Vater and into the second portion of the duodenum. This axial contrast enhanced CT demonstrates a 2.7-cm pancreatic psueudoaneurysm (arrow in Figure 71-1) in the pancreatic neck surrounded by a severely inflamed pancreas.

This condition is predominantly observed in males and seems to occur more commonly with chronic alcohol use as a complication of acute or chronic pancreatitis with rupture of a pseudoaneurysm or erosion of a pseudocyst through an adjacent arterial wall. The bleeding can be intermittent as coagulation of the blood may temporarily tamponade the problem. However, as the clot dissolves, then massive bleeding can resume. There can be accompaniment of increased pain with hyperamylasemia due to the increased pancreatic intraductal pressure causing distention.

Other causes of this condition include pancreatic tumor erosion into the pancreatic duct, or as a direct result from an iatrogenic complication after a therapeutic manipulation of the pancreatic duct with ERCP. Blunt or abdominal trauma is another rare etiology of hemosuccus pancreaticus.

After resuscitation and rapid diagnosis, the mainstay of treatment involves mesenteric angiographic embolization, which is successful in most cases. You can't just sit on this since there is a high mortality rate at greater than 90% with supportive care and observation alone. So, you will need to give your interventional radiologist a call. When angiographic means are unsuccessful, surgical therapy with resection and ligation of the bleeding vessel may then be needed.

Why Might This Be Tested? The name of this condition just sounds so cool. Plus, it's in Latin. We know that the importance in Board review correlates directly with anything in Latin. Just think about it: Esophagitis dissecans; dysphagia lusoria; acanthosis nigricans; pyoderma gangrenosum; pseudoxanthoma elasticum; hidradenitis suppurativa; pneumatosis intestinalis; colitis cystica profunda; etc. These are Board review classics. And all in Latin. Know 'em! (They are covered in one place or another throughout the *Acing* series.)

> ### Here's the Point! 1
>
> **GI bleed + Pancreatitis + Pseudoaneurysm + No mucosal abnormalities on EGD → Hemosuccus pancreaticus**

> ### Here's the Point! 2
>
> **Hemosuccus pancreaticus treatment → Mesenteric angiography with embolization**

Vignette 72: Tic or Treat?

An 81-year-old woman is admitted to the hospital due to "having severe gas attacks again." She had a cholecystectomy a few years ago and has now been admitted 4 times in the past 2 years with episodic cholangitis and pancreatitis. However, her workup has been negative and each episode resolved with antibiotics. She had an abdominal ultrasound and CT scan which were unremarkable. MRCP is now performed and is also unremarkable. Her abdominal pain resolves and on hospital day 3, labs return to normal including liver tests and lipase. Duodenoscopy is performed and the image is provided below (Figure 72-1).

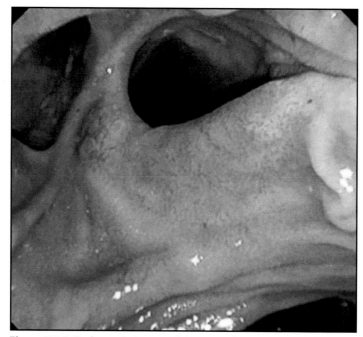

Figure 72-1. Endoscopic image of the ampullary region in the second portion of the duodenum.

▶ *What is the diagnosis?*

Vignette 72: Answer

This is Lemmel syndrome, which is a condition marked by recurrent episodes of cholangitis and pancreatitis due to episodic ampullary obstruction from a periampullary or juxtapapillary duodenal diverticulum. With this clinical presentation, there would be concern for ampullary adenoma or malignancy. Thus, the duodenoscopy was performed. The duodenum is the second most common site of diverticula formation in the gastrointestinal tract (you already knew that the colon was the most common site). Within the duodenum, the majority of diverticula are in the periampullary region. The mechanism of disease seems to be mechanical with enterolith or bezoar periodically getting impacted within the diverticulum leading to diverticulitis and resultant obstruction of the adjacent papilla which can lead to cholangitis or pancreatitis. Check out that endoscopic image again—you can see some residue still in there. Biliary stasis can then even lead to choledocholithiasis. It has also been theorized that the diverticulum can predispose patients to having an incompetent sphincter of Oddi, which may allow enteral contents to reflux into the papilla and produce intermittent cholangitis or pancreatitis. But the exact mechanism of this syndrome is poorly understood. We do know that the older you get, the more likely you will develop a periampullary diverticulum. Most patients with periampullary diverticula remain asymptomatic and require no endoscopic therapy. However, the plan of therapy here in this symptomatic patient would be ERCP with sphincterotomy to prevent recurrent disease. Contrary to popular belief, biliary cannulation has a similar success and complication rate in patients with a periampullary diverticulum compared to those without. Therefore, ERCP with sphincterotomy can be safely performed and would be beneficial in this case to help prevent further episodes of cholangitis or pancreatitis.

Why Might This Be Tested? Our population is getting older and you will be seeing periampullary diverticula more often. Although most remain asymptomatic, it is important to be cognizant of the potential consequences.

By the way, we named this "Tic or Treat" because the picture looks like a Jack-o'-Lantern (See it? Figure 72-2). Or is it Jack-o'-Lemmel? Just remember that if you eat lots of lemon (or Lemmel) Halloween candy it will give you gas. Then think about tics in the duodenum. (How's that for ridiculous?)

Figure 72-2. Best figure you've ever seen in a textbook.

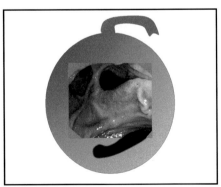

Here's the Point!

Recurrent cholangitis with negative imaging → Duodenoscopy to look at the ampulla for adenoma or periampullary diverticulum

Vignette 73: Oily Oozing

A 60-year-old man has had painful skin nodules for the past 6 months. He was seen by his dermatologist who treated with systemic steroids for presumed erythema nodosum, but there was no improvement. In addition, he has noticed a brownish oily discharge from some of these skin lesions. He reports an unintentional 25-lb weight loss without abdominal pain or nausea or vomiting. Serum laboratory tests are notable for lipase = 11,200 U/L. An abdominal CT scan is performed and shows a large 10-cm necrotic mass in the tail of the pancreas. A subsequent CT-guided biopsy of the pancreatic mass is performed, shown below in Figure 73-1.

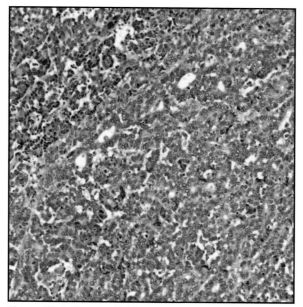

Figure 73-1. Pancreatic biopsy specimen. (Reprinted with permission from Vaidehi Avadhani, MD, Emory University.)

▶ *What is the diagnosis?*

Vignette 73: Answer

This is acinar cell carcinoma of the pancreas. The markedly elevated lipase levels are due to the tumor cells producing the excessive pancreatic enzymes; this is sometimes referred to as "lipase hypersecretion syndrome." This in turn, leads to peripheral fat necrosis with lipolysis leading to oozing of oily brown-colored discharge from the subcutaneous nodules (dissolving fat—pretty gnarly...). Polyarthralgias can accompany these skin lesions, also known as pancreatic panniculitis, which can be misdiagnosed as erythema nodosum. By the way, do you remember the differential of erythema nodosum? Look at the IBD *Acing* book for more on that.

Pancreatic panniculitis is more commonly seen with either acute or chronic pancreatitis, where patients will have abdominal pain. However, these subcutaneous nodules often precede other clinical symptoms when they are associated with acinar cell carcinoma of the pancreas. Thus, patients often may not have abdominal pain or anorexia by the time of diagnosis. In fact, the tumors are typically large at the time of diagnosis as in this case. Acinar cell carcinoma is quite rare and accounts for only 1% of all exocrine pancreatic malignancies; whereas, pancreatic ductal adenocarcinoma accounts for approximately 85%.

The histology (take a close look at that micrograph) of acinar cell carcinoma of the pancreas shows the acinar structure with round monotonous nuclei and a granular cytoplasm without much of a fibrous stroma, which contrasts the fibrosis commonly seen in pancreatic ductal adenocarcinoma. Therefore, proper utilization of a microscope should be able to differentiate these malignancies without much difficulty. Acinar cell carcinoma tends to be a more indolent disease and more often resectable at diagnosis, as opposed to ductal adenocarcinoma. Upon resection of the tumor, lipase levels typically return to normal and the skin lesions regress.

Why Might This Be Tested? Since most pancreatic cancers are ductal adenocarcinoma, this could be a misdirection type of play (a no-look pass) where you are led towards the more common, but incorrect diagnosis. This is a good reminder to stay focused and pay attention (always keep your eye on the ball) during the exam. It is also worthwhile to know some basic histology.

Here's the Point!

Painful cutaneous nodules + Elevated lipase + Large pancreatic tumor → Acinar cell carcinoma of the pancreas

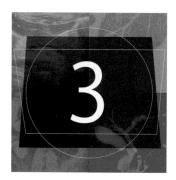

BOARD REVIEW
"CLINICAL THRESHOLD VALUES"

There are some factlets that you just have to know for Board review. To prepare for the test, it's good to memorize some numerical threshold values, like: *"Sphincter of Oddi manometry is considered abnormal when the nadir pressure is sustainably above 40 mm Hg in both leads across multiple stations"* or *"HIDA scan suggests biliary dyskinesia when the gallbladder ejection fraction falls below 40%."*

These have been highlighted throughout the book. What follows is a "one-stop shop" for all these little numerical facts. These are presented by increasing numerical order—not by a rational taxonomy. So, the resulting list will seem like a pretty random hodgepodge, which is the point. Exam questions are random, too, so just go with the flow.

1 mm = Normal bile duct diameter in elderly subjects increases 1 mm per decade of life—important to know so you are not fooled by seeming duct dilation in an otherwise healthy older person.

2 to 3 cm = So long as an ampullary adenoma is smaller than this size, and assuming there are no lymph nodes on imaging or extension of the tumor into the ductal systems on EUS, endoscopic ampullectomy remains a treatment option.

3 mm = Normal gallbladder wall thickness is at, or below, this width.

3x ULN = When lipase exceeds this threshold in the setting of pancreatitis from hypertriglyceridemia, consider initiating plasma exchange (also when there is hypocalcemia, lactic acidosis, and signs of organ dysfunction).

3x ULN = Amylase level is above this threshold to meet laboratory criteria for post-ERCP pancreatitis.

Spiegel BMR, Karsan HA.
Acing the Pancreaticobiliary Questions on the GI Board Exam:
The Ultimate Crunch-Time Resource (pp 137-138).
© 2018 Taylor & Francis Group.

3-2-1 Rule = Normal pancreatic duct diameter is up to 3 mm in the head, 2 mm in the body, and 1 mm in the tail of the pancreas.

6 mm = Normal bile duct diameter in patients who have not undergone cholecystectomy is at, or below, this threshold.

7 mm = Puestow operation indicated in chronic calcific pancreatitis with a pancreatic duct of this diameter or larger.

11.5 French = Largest plastic biliary stent is this diameter (~4 mm). (Related thresholds: 3 French is 1 mm: largest biliary SEMS is 10 mm in diameter.)

20% = In normal healthy patients, more than this percentage of pancreatic function is required to maintain clinically adequate exocrine and endocrine function.

30% = If more than this amount of the pancreatic parenchyma is nonviable in the setting of pancreatitis, then it is considered to be necrotizing pancreatitis.

40 mm Hg = Sphincter of Oddi manometry is considered abnormal when the nadir pressure is sustainably above this pressure in both leads across multiple stations.

40% = HIDA scan results suggest biliary dyskinesia when the gallbladder ejection fraction falls below this value in a patient with biliary colic.

50 = If the stool osmolar gap (290 – 2[Na+K]) is lower than this in a patient with diarrhea, then the mechanism is most likely secretory diarrhea. (Related threshold: If the stool osmolar gap is above 125 mOsm/kg, then osmotic diarrhea is suggested.)

60 mmol/L = Sweat chloride is typically at, or above, this level in cystic fibrosis.

75 pg/mL = VIP above this threshold is suggestive of VIPoma.

90% = Clinically significant fat and protein deficiencies do not typically occur until more than this percentage of pancreatic function is lost.

192 ng/mL = CEA above this threshold in pancreatic cyst fluid helps to differentiate a mucinous from a nonmucinous neoplasm. However, CEA level in pancreatic cyst fluid is not predictive of malignancy.

200 mcg/g = Fecal elastase below this threshold suggests pancreatic exocrine insufficiency. (Related threshold: Fecal elastase < 100 mcg/g indicates severe pancreatic exocrine insufficiency.)

280 mg/dL = Serum IgG4 above this level is suggestive of autoimmune pancreatitis. (Serum IgG4 is normally below 140 mg/dL.)

500 g/dL = Initiate intravenous insulin for hypertriglyceridemia-induced pancreatitis when serum blood glucose is above this threshold.

500 pg/mL = Glucagon above this threshold is suggestive of glucagonoma.

1000 mg/dL = Hypertriglyceridemina is considered a risk factor for pancreatitis when levels are above this value. Also, consider therapeutic plasma exchange for acute pancreatitis when serum triglycerides exceed this threshold.

10,000 units/kg/day = Supplemental lipase dose should not exceed this threshold or else risk complications like colonic strictures. (Related threshold: Should also not exceed 2500 units/kg/meal.)

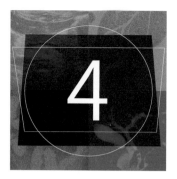

"CRUNCH-TIME" SELF-TEST—
TIME TO GET YOUR GAME ON

This is a rapid-fire "crunch-time" self-test. The questions in this test are based on the "Here's the Point!" bullet points from each of the vignettes in the preceding section. These represent the distilled essence of Board review vignettes, so know them well. As you read each one-liner, write in the diagnosis in the corresponding blank line. Really... just actively write it in right there on the page. For these questions, you'll need to know the diagnosis first to know what to do next. So, this is a bottom-line test of your basic diagnostic capabilities for the "tough stuff" in Board review. Few of these are true "gimmies." If you've carefully studied the vignettes up to this point, then this should be a relative snap—and should reaffirm that you're well on your way to acing the "tough stuff." Some of these are stand-alone questions that do not have a corresponding vignette in the book. Once you're done, check with the answer key and score yourself according to the interpretation guide starting on page 159, and try not to cheat too much—just write down your best guess prior to checking the answer, and then add up all the correct answers you get once you're done (no partial credit!). If you cheat your way through this test, then you won't know how you did and won't be able to interpret your score per the guide starting on page 159. If you're in crunch time, then once you're done, make sure to look up the corresponding vignettes for each of the items you got wrong, and study those vignettes carefully to fill in your knowledge gaps.

Okay, let's do this.

Spiegel BMR, Karsan HA.
Acing the Pancreaticobiliary Questions on the GI Board Exam:
The Ultimate Crunch-Time Resource (pp 139-152).
© 2018 Taylor & Francis Group.

Question 1. Acute pancreatitis + xanthomas + diabetes.

▶ Diagnosis _____

Question 2. Pancreatic cyst + microcystic ("honeycomb") appearance.

▶ Diagnosis _____

Question 3. Flushing + secretory diarrhea + profound hypochlorhydria.

▶ Diagnosis _____

Question 4. What's this?

▶ _____

Questions 5-6. A patient with FAP develops acute pancreatitis. Name 2 different causes of pancreatitis related to a patient with FAP.

▶ Cause #1 _____
▶ Cause #2 _____

Question 7. What liver tumor typically causes capsular retraction instead of a bulge?

▶ Diagnosis _____

Question 8. High-dose pancreatic enzyme supplements + colonic obstruction.

▶ Diagnosis _____

Questions 9-12. Name 4 things that can cause both gynecomastia and pancreatitis.
► Thing #1 _____
► Thing #2 _____
► Thing #3 _____
► Thing #4 _____

Question 13. What's this?

► _____

Question 14. UTI + commonly prescribed antibiotic + acute pancreatitis.
► Most likely culprit _____

Question 15. Chronic diarrhea + anemia + papillary stenosis + recurrent pancreatitis + normal CD4 count.
► Diagnosis _____

Questions 16-23. Name 8 risk factors for post-ERCP pancreatitis.
► Risk factor _____
► Risk factor _____
► Risk factor _____
► Risk factor _____
► Risk factor _____
► Risk factor _____
► Risk factor _____
► Risk factor _____

Questions 24-26. What is the generally preferred intravenous fluid solution for acute pancreatitis? Why? In what situation is it not preferred?
► Preferred solution _____
► Why it's preferred _____
► When it *isn't* preferred _____

Questions 27-29. Child with chronic cholestasis + cardiac abnormalities + "butterfy vertebrae" + posterior embryotoxon of the eye + dysmorphic facies + ductopenia on liver biopsy.

▶ Diagnosis _____

▶ Autosomal dominant or recessive _____

▶ Mutated gene _____

Question 30. "Sausage shaped" pancreas + recurrent pancreatitis.

▶ Diagnosis _____

Question 31. Seizure disorder + acute pancreatitis.

▶ Diagnosis _____

Question 32. What's this?

▶ _____

Question 33. A pregnant woman develops significant hypertriglyceridemia and acute pancreatitis. What underlying condition might she have?

▶ Diagnosis _____

Question 34. What is the preferred way to manage WOPN in a clinically unstable patient?

▶ Management _____

Question 35. Obstructive jaundice + gallstone in cystic duct compressing common hepatic duct.

▶ Diagnosis _____

Question 36. Beyond fluid resuscitation and supportive care, what specific therapy should be considered for progression of acute pancreatitis with hypertriglyceridemia >1000 mg/dL?

▶ Treatment _____

Questions 37-38. Recurrent idiopathic pancreatitis + double duct sign on MRCP + no pancreatic mass on MRI.

▶ What test do you perform? _____
▶ What are you looking for? _____

Question 39. What's this?

▶ _____

Question 40. What is the first-line treatment for an uncomplicated choledochocele?

▶ Treatment _____

Questions 41-43. What action do you take with cholecystitis with a low risk of retained stone? How about a medium risk? And high risk?

▶ Low risk _____
▶ Medium risk _____
▶ High risk _____

Question 44. PSC + acute jaundice + weight loss + new dominant stricture.

▶ Suspected diagnosis _____

Questions 45-47. Name 3 antihypertensive medications that can cause pancreatitis.

▶ Medication #1 _____
▶ Medication #2 _____
▶ Medication #3 _____

Questions 48-50. What is the most common congenital pancreatic abnormality? About what percentage of the population has this condition? What other congenital pancreatic abnormality is this associated with?

▶ Diagnosis _____

▶ Percentage of population _____

▶ Associated congenital pancreatic abnormality _____

Question 51. Recent cholecystectomy + right upper quadrant pain + right upper quadrant fluid collection.

▶ Diagnosis _____

Question 52. Is surgery indicated for an asymptomatic pseudocyst >6 cm that persists >6 weeks after a bout of acute pancreatitis?

▶ Yes / No _____

Question 53. What is the preferred way to manage a symptomatic WOPN in a clinically stable patient without a pseudoaneurysm?

▶ Management _____

Questions 54-56. Name 3 inflammatory bowel disease meds that can cause pancreatitis.

▶ Medication #1 _____

▶ Medication #2 _____

▶ Medication #3 _____

Questions 57-59. What are the top 3 causes of pancreatitis, in order?

▶ Cause #1 _____

▶ Cause #2 _____

▶ Cause #3 _____

Question 60. What's this?

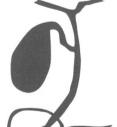

▶ _____

Question 61. Preferred treatment of malignant biliary obstruction with >3-month expected survival.

▶ Treatment _____

Questions 62-64. Name 3 contraindications to surgery in the setting of a pancreatic mass.

▶ Contraindication #1 _____
▶ Contraindication #2 _____
▶ Contraindication #3 _____

Question 65. Is it good to "acinarize" the pancreas on an ERCP pancreatogram?

▶ Yes / No _____

Question 66. What's this?

▶ _____

Questions 67-68. WOPN + acute abdominal pain + pallor + hypotension.

▶ Diagnosis _____
▶ Treatment _____

Questions 69-70. Pancreatitis + isolated gastric varices.

▶ Diagnosis _____
▶ Definitive management if varices bleed _____

Questions 71-73. Family history of melanoma + family history of pancreatic cancer + multiple dysplastic nevi.

▶ Diagnosis _____
▶ Autosomal dominant or recessive _____
▶ Gene mutation _____

Question 74. A benign little volcano-looking thing in the antrum.

▶ Diagnosis _____

Question 75. Most likely pancreatic cyst in a young woman.

▶ Diagnosis _____

Question 76. Name a medicine that you probably haven't prescribed for years but is very important for GI Board review due to significant pancreatic and hepatic side effects.

▶ Medicine _____

Question 77. Pancreatic cyst + gelatinous ooze from ampulla.

▶ Diagnosis _____

Question 78. Pancreatic cyst + "cluster of grapes" appearance on imaging.

▶ Diagnosis _____

Question 79. Hypomelanotic macule + cardiac rhabdomyoma + renal angiolipoma + insulinoma.

▶ Diagnosis _____

Question 80. Middle-aged female + pancreatic cyst in tail + fluid analysis with low amylase and high CEA.

▶ Diagnosis _____

Question 81. What tumor is associated with annular pancreas?

▶ Diagnosis _____

Question 82. Pancreatic cyst + fish mouth ampulla.

▶ Diagnosis _____

Questions 83-89. Gene mix 'n' match. On the left is a set of genetic conditions that can also affect the pancreas. One the right are gene mutations. Draw a line from each condition to the correct gene.

Peutz-Jeghers syndrome   CDKN2A

Autosomal dominant hereditary pancreatitis   DNA mismatch repair genes

FAMMM syndrome   STK11

Lynch syndrome   BRCA2

Autosomal recessive hereditary pancreatitis   CFTR

Hereditary breast cancer   SPINK1

Cystic fibrosis   PRSS-1

Question 90. Recurrent pancreatitis + periductal lymphoplasmacytic infiltrate, obliterative phlebitis, and acinar fibrosis on biopsy.

▶ Diagnosis _____

Question 91. Liver transplant for nonHCV indication + jaundice and cholestasis + patent hepatic artery on ultrasound.

▶ Primary concern _____

Question 92. What is the preferred way to manage WOPN in a clinically stable patient with a pseudoaneurysm?

▶ Management _____

Question 93. Large biliary sphincterotomy or precut papillotomy + post-ERCP abdominal pain + normal serum lipase.

▶ What are you most concerned about? _____

Question 94. Young adult + chronic pancreatitis + multiple family members with pancreatic cancer.

▶ Diagnosis _____

Question 95. Older diabetic man + fever + right upper quadrant crepitus and pain + "Champagne sign" on ultrasonography.

▶ Diagnosis _____

Question 96. What's this?

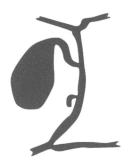

▶ _____

Questions 97-100. For each condition listed, indicate whether UCDA can help reduce disease
progression.
▶ PBC (yes / no)_____
▶ PSC (yes / no)_____
▶ Recurrent pyogenic cholangitis (yes / no) _____
▶ Cholestasis of cystic fibrosis (yes / no) _____

Question 101. Young person with pancreatic insufficiency + chronic neutropenia + short
stature.
▶ Diagnosis _____

Questions 102-103. A critically ill patient has fever, leukocytosis, gallbladder wall thickening,
and pericholecystic fluid but no gallstones. What is the diagnosis and, other
than starting antibiotics, how else should you treat?
▶ Diagnosis _____
▶ Treatment_____

Question 104. Name of the rash found in glucagonoma.
▶ Diagnosis _____

Questions 105-106. What are the top 2 primary cancers that metastasizes to the pancreas?
▶ Cancer #1 _____
▶ Cancer #2 _____

Question 107. Parathyroid adenoma + Pituitary adenoma + Pancreatic neuroendocrine tumor.
▶ Diagnosis _____

Question 108. What type of PNET is associated with neurofibromatosis?
▶ Diagnosis _____

Questions 109-110. Name 2 antiarrhythmic medications that can cause pancreatitis.
▶ Medication #1 _____
▶ Medication #2 _____

Questions 111-112. Name 2 things that can appear anechoic in the third ultrasonographic layer of the stomach.
▶ Thing #1_____
▶ Thing #2_____

Question 113. Which of these biliary cysts is least worrisome: type I, type II, type III, type IV, type V?
▶ Least worrisome cyst _____

Question 114. "Double bubble sign."
▶ Diagnosis _____

Question 115. Acute cardiovascular or neurologic collapse during ERCP + no free air on fluoroscopy.
▶ What are you most worried about? _____

Question 116. What's the most durable treatment for chronic calcific pancreatitis with a dilated pancreatic duct?
▶ Treatment _____

Question 117. Obstruction of the portal vein with collaterals causing extrinsic bile duct obstruction.
▶ Diagnosis _____

Question 118. What is the sole artery that supplies the bile duct?
▶ Name of artery_____

Question 119. How do you manage a patient with a large bile duct stone and ascending cholangitis who is on anticoagulation?
▶ Management _____

Question 120. Patient with hepatitis C cirrhosis undergoes a liver transplant, and later develops rapidly progressive hepatitis, graft failure, and cholestasis.

▶ Diagnosis _____

Question 121. Hemangioblastoma + renal cell carcinoma + pheochromocytoma + pancreatic tumor.

▶ Diagnosis _____

Question 122. What's this?

▶ _____

Question 123. Pneumobilia + small bowel obstruction + gallstone in right iliac fossa.

▶ Diagnosis _____

Question 124. Inflammatory bowel disease + recurrent pancreatitis + granulocytic epithelial lesion in pancreatic duct + minimal IgG4-positive cells in pancreatic parenchyma biopsy.

▶ Diagnosis _____

Question 125. Name the condition which causes a "strawberry" appearance of gross examination of the gallbladder.

▶ Diagnosis _____

Questions 126-127. Name 2 malignancies associated with anomalous panc-bil junction.

▶ Cancer #1 _____
▶ Cancer #2 _____

Questions 128-133. What type of gallstone is most likely for each of these conditions?

▶ Sickle cell anemia_____

▶ Recurrent pyogenic cholangitis _____

▶ Rapid weight loss _____

▶ Neurofibromatosis_____

▶ Longstanding TPN _____

▶ Cirrhosis _____

Questions 134-135. Pancreatic cyst + microcystic ("honeycomb") appearance.

▶ Diagnosis _____

▶ Malignant potential (high / low)_____

Questions 136-137. Asian woman + cholecystitis + hypoechoic nodules in gallbladder wall.

▶ Diagnosis _____

▶ Is this a premalignant lesion? _____

Question 138. Diarrhea + Dermatitis + Diabetes + Weight Loss.

▶ Diagnosis _____

Question 139. Gallbladder wall calcification.

▶ Diagnosis _____

Question 140. What's the most common extrapancreatic manifestation of type 1 autoimmune pancreatitis?

▶ Treatment _____

Question 141. Jaundice after cholecystectomy + no proximal bile duct opacification on ERCP + surgical clip in vicinity of bile duct.

▶ Diagnosis _____

Question 142. What biliary lesion does celiac disease have in common with AIDS cholangiopathy?

▶ Name of lesion _____

Question 143. What ductal abnormality is often seen alongside type I biliary cysts?

▶ Diagnosis _____

Question 144. Billroth II anatomy + post-ERCP abdominal pain + normal lipase + free air
          under the diaphragm.

▶ Where is the perforation most likely (be specific)?_____

Question 145. Most common cause of pancreatitis in children?

▶ Diagnosis _____

Questions 146-147. Epigastric pain + succussion splash + calcification in pylorus. Other than
          saying this is gallstone ileus, which it is, what specifically led to this syn-
          drome, and what's it called?

▶ Cause of syndrome _____
▶ Name of syndrome _____

Question 148. Pancreatic tumor + peripheral fat necrosis.

▶ Diagnosis _____

Question 149. Pancreatic tumor + weight gain.

▶ Diagnosis _____

Question 150. Elderly patient + recurrent cholangitis and pancreatitis + normal MRCP +
          duodenoscopy shows no ampullary adenoma.

▶ Diagnosis _____

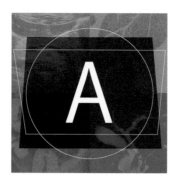

Appendix A
Answers to "Crunch-Time" Self-Test

1. Hypertriglyceridemia-induced pancreatitis
2. Serous cystadenoma
3. VIPoma
4. Type III biliary cyst (aka choledochocele)
5. Ampullary adenoma
6. Sulindac
7. Cholangiocarcinoma
8. Fibrosing colonopathy from pancreatic enzymes
9. Cannabis
10. Anabolic steroids
11. Cimetidine
12. Alcohol
13. Type I biliary cyst
14. Trimethoprim-sulfamethoxazole
15. Celiac disease

Spiegel BMR, Karsan HA.
Acing the Pancreaticobiliary Questions on the GI Board Exam:
The Ultimate Crunch-Time Resource (pp 153-157).
© 2018 Taylor & Francis Group.

16. Suspected sphincter of Oddi dysfunction

17. Female gender

18. Younger (< 50 years old)

19. Difficult cannulation

20. Acinarization with pancreatic duct injection

21. Messing with sphincter: ampullectomy, balloon dilation of sphincter

22. Inexperienced endoscopist

23. Previous history of pancreatitis

24. Lactated Ringer's solution

25. More pH balanced vs saline; less likely to activate trypsinogen and cause hyperchloremic metabolic acidosis

26. Hypercalcemia-induced pancreatitis

27. Alagille syndrome (Nope, wasn't in the book! But this should be enough to know.)

28. Autosomal dominant

29. Associated with mutation in JAG1 gene

30. Autoimmune pancreatitis

31. Valproic acid

32. Anomalous panc-bil junction

33. Type IV familial hyperlipidemia (high VLDL)

34. Surgical necrosectomy

35. Mirizzi's syndrome

36. Plasma exchange

37. Side-viewing duodenoscopy of ampulla

38. Ampullary tumor or periampullary abnormality

39. Pancreas divisum

40. Sphincterotomy

41. Surgery without preop ERCP

42. Preop EUS or MRCP

43. Preop ERCP

44. Cholangiocarcinoma

45. Furosemide

46. Hydrocholorothiazide

47. Enalapril (also Losartan)

48. Pancreas divium

49. 7%

50. Annular pancreas

51. Biloma

52. Nope

53. Endoscopic (or possibly percutaneous) necrosectomy

54. Azathioprine

55. Mesalamine

56. Steroids

57. Alcohol

58. Gallstones

59. Hypertriglyceridemia

60. Annular pancreas

61. Self-expanding metal stent

62. Poor surgical candidate (obviously…)

63. Vascular involvement (especially if > 180° around major vessel)

64. Metastatic spread

65. Nope. That's no good.

66. Double duct sign

67. Pseudoaneurysm rupture

68. Angiography with embolization by interventional radiologist or surgery

69. Splenic vein thrombosis

70. Splenectomy

71. FAMMM syndrome (familial atypical multiple mole melanoma syndrome)

72. Autosomal dominant

73. CDKN2A on chromosome 9

74. Pancreatic rest (aka heterotopic pancreas)

75. Solid pseudopapillary neoplasm

76. Valproic acid! (and others…)

77. Main-duct intraductal papillary mucinous neoplasm (IPMN)

78. Branch-duct IPMN

79. Tuberous sclerosis

80. Mucinous cystic neoplasm

81. Ampullary adenoma

82. Yep, main-duct IPMN again

83. Peutz Jeghers → STK11

84. Autosomal dominant hereditary pancreatitis → PRSS-1

85. FAMMM → CDKN2A

86. Lynch syndrome → DNA mismatch repair genes

87. Autosomal recessive hereditary pancreatitis → SPINK1

88. Hereditary breast cancer → BRCA2

89. Cystic fibrosis → CFTR

90. Type 1 autoimmune pancreatitis

91. Anastomotic biliary stricture

92. Surgical necrosectomy (not endoscopic or percutaneous)

93. Retroperitoneal perforation

94. PRSS-1 gene mutation

95. Emphysematous cholecystitis

96. Type II biliary cyst

97. Yes

98. No

99. No

100. Yes

101. Shwachman-Diamond Syndrome (SDS). Nope, this wasn't in the book. Here's what you need to know: SDS is an autosomal recessive disease and the second most common cause of pancreatic insufficiency in kids behind cystic fibrosis. These patients are at increased risk of developing myelodysplastic syndrome and they have skeletal abnormalities and other findings described in the question stem.

102. Acalculous cholecystitis

103. Place cholecystostomy tube

104. Necrolytic migratory erythema

105. Renal cell cancer (#1)

106. Melanoma (#2)

107. Multiple endocrine neoplasia (MEN) I

108. Somatostatinoma

109. Amiodarone

110. Procainamide

111. Gastric varices

112. Duplication cyst

113. Type 3

114. Annular pancreas (wasn't thinking about pyloric hypertrophy, the other "double bubble")

115. Suspect air embolus

116. Puestow procedure (lateral pancreaticojejunostomy)

117. Portal biliopathy

118. Hepatic artery

119. Plastic biliary stent; no sphincterotomy

120. Fibrosing cholestatic hepatitis

121. von Hippel-Lindau

122. Recurrent pyogenic cholangitis

123. Gallstone ileus

124. Type 2 autoimmune pancreatitis

125. Cholesterolosis of gallbladder

126. Cholangiocarcinoma

127. Gallbladder cancer

128. Black pigment stone

129. Brown pigment or "mixed" stone

130. Cholesterol stone

131. Cholesterol stone (from somatostatinoma-induced biliary dyskinesia)

132. Cholesterol stone

133. Black pigment stone

134. Serous cystadenoma

135. Low

136. Xanthogranulomatous cholecystitis

137. No, not premalignant

138. Glucagonoma

139. Porcelain gallbladder

140. Sclerosing cholangitis

141. Bile duct transection... ☹

142. Papillary stenosis

143. APBJ

144. Lateral wall of duodenum

145. Trauma

146. Cholecystogastric fistula with gastric outlet obstruction due to a large gallstone

147. Bouveret syndrome

148. Acinar cell carcinoma

149. Insulinoma (eating to counteract hypoglycemia)

150. Lemmel syndrome (periampullary diverticulum)

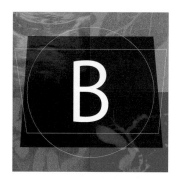

Appendix B
"Crunch-Time" Self-Test
Scoring Guide

150 correct: You cheated.

140-149:   You still cheated.

135-139:   Impossible to believe.

130-134:   Either you cheated, or you're a monster diagnostician ready to crush the Boards.

125-129:   Assuming you didn't cheat, that was a crazy good performance.

120-124:   Outstanding performance—way above the mean.

115-119:   Pretty darn tremendous.

110-114:   Highly respectable—well above average for this level of difficulty.

105-109:   Good work—you're definitely ahead of the curve.

100-104:   You're doing fine—a good effort.

95-99:   Don't despair—these are hard, and you hung in well.

90-94:   Not terrible, but you need to start fine-tuning the rough spots.

85-89:   Could be better.

80-84:   Look in the mirror. Then say, "I know I can do better. Let's kick this up a notch."

Spiegel BMR, Karsan HA.
Acing the Pancreaticobiliary Questions on the GI Board Exam:
The Ultimate Crunch-Time Resource (pp 159-160).
© 2018 Taylor & Francis Group.

75-79:   You're in the 50% range now—mediocre.

70-74:   Not good enough—below average.

65-69:   These are tough, but you're below the curve.

60-64:   Inadequate knowledge base. You're in jeopardy of not passing the exam.

55-59:   Yikes.

50-54:   Double yikes.

< 50:   Wait a while before taking the exam. You've got a way to go.

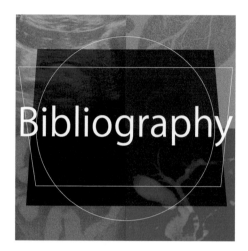

Bibliography

Adler DG, Qureshi W, Davila R, et al. The role of endoscopy in ampullary and duodenal adenomas. *Gastrointest Endosc.* 2006;64(6):849-854.

Ahmed Ali U, Pahlplatz JM, Nealon WH, et al. Endoscopic or surgical intervention for painful bstructive chronic pancreatitis. *Cochrane Database Syst Rev.* 2015;19:3.

Al-Omran M, Albalawi ZH, Tashkandi MF, et al. Enteral versus parenteral nutrition for acute pancreatitis. *Cochrane Database Syst Rev.* 2010;(1):CD002837.

Anderson MA, Fisher L, Jain R, et al. Complications of ERCP. *Gastrointest Endosc.* 2012;75(3):467-473.

Badalov N, Baradarian R, Iswara K, Li J, Steniberg W, Tenner S. Drug-induced acute pancreatitis: an evidence-based review. *Clin Gastroenterol Hepatol.* 2007;5(6):648-661.

Bakker OJ, van Santvoort HC, van Brunschot S, et al. Endoscopic transgastric vs surgical necrosectomy for infected necrotizing pancreatitis: a randomized trial. *JAMA.* 2012;307(10):1053-1061.

Basha J, Appasani S, Vaiphei K, et al. Celiac disease presenting as recurrent pancreatitis and pseudocyst. *JOP.* 2012;13(5):533-535.

Brown A, Hughes M, Tenner S, Banks PA. Does pancreatic enzyme supplementation reduce pain in patients with chronic pancreatitis: a meta-analysis. *Am J Gastroenterol.* 1997;92(11):2032-2035.

Cahen DL, Gouma DJ, Laramée P, et al. Long-term outcomes of endoscopic vs surgical drainage of the pancreatic duct in patients with chronic pancreatitis. *Gastroenterology.* 2011;141(5):1690-1695.

Chapman MH, Webster GJ, Bannoo S, Johnson GJ, Wittmann J, Pereira SP. Cholangiocarcinoma and dominant strictures in patients with primary sclerosing cholangitis: a 25-year single-centre experience. *Eur J Gastroenterol Hepatol.* 2012;24(9):1051-1058.

Chapman R, Fevery J, Kalloo A, et al. Diagnosis and management of primary sclerosing cholangitis. *Hepatology.* 2010;51(2):660-678.

Chaudary P. Acinar Cell Carcinoma of the Pancreas: A Literature Review and Update. *Indian J Surg.* 2015;77(3):226-231.

Chiang TH, Lee YC, Chiu HM, Huang SP, Lin JT, Wang HP. Endoscopic therapeutics for patients with cholangitis caused by the juxtapapillary duodenal diverticulum. *Hepatogastroenterology.* 2006;53(70):501-505.

Chun KA, Ha HK, Yu ES, et al. Xanthogranulomatous cholecystitis: CT features with emphasis on differentiation from gallbladder carcinoma. *Radiology.* 1997;203(1):93-97.

Cohen J, Sawhney MS, Pleskow DK, et al. Double-duct sign in the era of endoscopic ultrasound: the prevalence of occult pancreaticobiliary malignancy. *Dig Dis Sci.* 2014;59(9):2280-2285.

Cotton PB, Durkalski V, Romagnuolo J, et al. Effect of endoscopic sphincterotomy for suspected sphincter of Oddi dysfunction on pain-related disability following cholecystectomy: the EPISOD randomized clinical trial. *JAMA.* 2014;311(20):2101-2109.

Ducarme G, Maire F, Chatel P, Luton D, Hammel P. Acute pancreatitis during pregnancy: a review. *J Perinatol.* 2014;34(2):87-94.

Egawa N, Anjiki H, Takuma K, Kamisawa T. Juxtapapillary duodenal diverticula and pancreaticobiliary disease. *Dig Surg.* 2010;27(2):105-109.

Fatma H, Mouna B, Leila M, Radhouane D, Taoufik N. Cannabis: a rare cause of acute pancreatitis. *Clin Res Hepatol Gastroenterol.* 2013;37(1):e24-25.

Finsterer J, Stollberger C, Bastovansky A. Cardiac and cerebral air embolism from endoscopic retrograde cholangio-pancreatography. *Eur J Gastroenterol Hepatol.* 2010;22(10):1157-1162.

Fogel EL, Sherman S. ERCP for gallstone pancreatitis. *N Engl J Med.* 2014;370(2):150-157.

Forns X, Charlton M, Denning J, et al. Sofosbuvir compassionate use program for patients with severe recurrent hepatitis C after liver transplantation. *Hepatology.* 2015;61:1485–1494.

Friedel D, Stavropoulos S, Iqbal S, Cappell MS. Gastrointestinal endoscopy in the pregnant woman. *World J Gastrointest Endosc.* 2014;6(5):156-167.

Grover S, Syngal S. Hereditary pancreatic cancer. *Gastroenterology.* 2010;139(4):1076-1080.

Habbe N, Langer P, Sina-Frey M, Bartsch DK. Familial pancreatic cancer syndromes. *Endocrinol Metab Clin North Am.* 2006;35(2):417-430.

Han B, Song ZF, Sun B. Hemosuccus pancreaticus: a rare cause of gastrointestinal bleeding. *Hepatobiliary Pancreat Dis Int.* 2012;11(5):479-488.

Holt AP, Thorburn D, Mirza D, Gunson B, Wong T, Haydon G. A prospective study of standardized nonsurgical therapy in the management of biliary anastomotic strictures complicating liver transplantation. *Transplantation.* 2007;84(7):857-863.

Jablonska B. Biliary cysts: etiology, diagnosis and management. *World J Gastroenterol.* 2012;18(35):4801-4810.

Kang HS, Hyun JJ, Kim SY, et al. Lemmel's syndrome, an unusual cause of abdominal pain and jaundice by impacted intradiverticular enterolith: case report. *J Korean Med Sci.* 2014;29(6):874-878.

Kanth R, Samji NS, Inaganti A, et al. Endotherapy in symptomatic pancreas divisum: a systematic review. *Pancreatology.* 2014;14(4):244-250.

Khalid A, Brugge W. ACG practice guidelines for the diagnosis and management of neoplastic pancreatic cysts. *Am J Gastroenterol.* 2007;102(10):2339-2349.

Kim HK, Lo SK. Endoscopic approach to the patient with benign or malignant ampullary lesions. *Gastrointest Endosc Clin N Am.* 2013;23(2):347-383.

Kunz PL, Reidy-Lagunes D, Anthony LB, et al. Consensus guidelines for the management and treatment of neuroendocrine tumors. *Pancreas.* 2013;42(4):557-577.

Laramée P, Wonderling D, Cahen DL, et al. Trial-based cost-effectiveness analysis comparing surgical and endoscopic drainage in patients with obstructive chronic pancreatitis. *BMJ Open.* 2013;3(9).

Lenhart DK, Balthazar EJ. MDCT of acute mild (nonnecrotizing) pancreatitis: abdominal complications and fate of fluid collections. *AJR Am J Roentgenol.* 2008;190(3):643-669.

Leroy V, Dumortier J, Coilly A, et al. Efficacy of sofosbuvir and daclatasvir in patients with fibrosing cholestatic hepatitis C after liver transplantation. *Clin Gastroenterol Hepatol.* 2015;13:1993–2001.

Liao Z, Gao R, Wang W, et al. A systematic review on endoscopic detection rate, endotherapy, and surgery for pancreas divisum. *Endoscopy.* 2009;41(5):439-444.

Lloyd-Still JD, Beno DW, Kimura RM. Cystic fibrosis colonopathy. *Curr Gastroenterol Rep.* 1999;1(3):231-237.

Lucey MR, Terrault N, Ojo L, et al. Long-term management of the successful adult liver transplant: 2012 practice guideline by the American Association for the Study of Liver Diseases and the American Society of Transplantation. *Liver Transpl.* 2013;19(1):3-26.

Luu MB, Deziel DJ. Unusual complications of gallstones. *Surg Clin North Am.* 2014;94(2):377-394.

Mahajani RV, Uzer MF. Cholangiopathy in HIV-infected patients. *Clin Liver Dis.* 1999;3(3):669-684.

Moayyedi PM, Lacy BE, Andrews CN, et al. ACG and CAG Clinical Guideline: Management of Dyspepsia. *Am J Gastroenterol.* 2017;112(7):988-1013.

Moss AC, Morris E, Leyden J, MacMathuna P. Do the benefits of metal stents justify the costs? A systematic review and meta-analysis of trials comparing endoscopic stents for malignant biliary obstruction. *Eur J Gastroenterol Hepatol.* 2007;19(12):1119-1124.

Moss AC, Morris E, Leyden J, MacMathuna P. Malignant distal biliary obstruction: a systematic review and meta-analysis of endoscopic and surgical bypass results. *Cancer Treat Rev.* 2007;33(2):213-221.

Nadkarni NA, Khanna S, Vege SS. Splanchnic venous thrombosis and pancreatitis. *Pancreas*. 2013;42(6):924-931.

Nally DM, Kelly EG, Clarke M, Ridgway P. Nasogastric nutrition is efficacious in severe acute pancreatitis: a systematic review and meta-analysis. *Br J Nutr*. 2014;112(11):1-10.

Nishida T, Kawai N, Yamaguchi S, Nishida Y. Submucosal tumors: comprehensive guide for the diagnosis and therapy of gastrointestinal submucosal tumors. *Dig Endosc*. 2013,25(5):479-489.

Nitsche CJ, Jamieson N, Lerch MM, Mayerle JV. Drug induced pancreatitis. *Best Pract Res Clin Gastroenterol*. 2010;24(2):143-155.

Ono M, Kamisawa T, Tu Y, Egawa N. MRCP and ERCP in Lemmel Syndrome. *JOP*. 2005;6(3):277-278.

O'Reilly DA, Malde DJ, Duncan T, Rao M, Filobbos R. Review of the diagnosis, classification and management of autoimmune pancreatitis. *World J Gastrointest Pathophysiol*. 2014;5(2):71-81.

Pang TC, Maher R, Gananadha S, Hugh TJ, Samra JS. Peripancreatic pseudoaneurysms: a management-based classification system. *Surg Endosc*. 2014;28(7):2027-2038.

Pfau PR, Banerjee S, Barth BA, et al. Sphincter of Oddi manometry. *Gastrointest Endosc*. 2011;74(6):1175-1180.

Rebours V, Boutron-Ruault MC, Schnee M, et al. The natural history of hereditary pancreatitis: a national series. *Gut*. 2009;58(1):97-103.

Robertson, MB, Choe KA, Joseph PM. Review of the abdominal manifestations of cystic fibrosis in the adult patient. *Radiographic*. 2006;26(3):679-690.

Sadr-Azodi O, Sanders DS, Murray JA, Ludvigsson JF. Patients with celiac disease have an increased risk for pancreatitis. *Clin Gastroenterol Hepatol*. 2012;10(10):1136-1142.

Scherer J, Singh VP, Pitchumoni CS, Yadav D. Issues in hypertriglyceridemic pancreatitis: an update. *J Clin Gastroenterol*. 2014;48(3):195-203.

Schnelldorfer T. Porcelain gallbladder: a benign process or concern for malignancy? *J Gastrointest Surg*. 2013;17(6):1161-1168.

Stewart L. Iatrogenic biliary injuries: identification, classification, and management. *Surg Clin North Am*. 2014;94(2):297-310.

Suraweera D, Sundaram V, Saab S. Treatment of hepatitis C virus infection in liver transplant recipients. *Gastroenterol Hepatol (N Y)*. 2016;12(1):23-30.

Tabrizian P, Newell P, Reiter BP, Heinmann TM. Successful multimodality treatment for hemosuccus pancreaticus. *Am J Gastroenterol*. 2009;104:1060.

Tenner S, Baillie J, DeWitt J, Vege SS, American College of Gastroenterology. American College of Gastroenterology guideline: management of acute pancreatitis. *Am J Gastroenterol*. 2013;108(9):1400-1416.

Tsuang W, Navaneethan U, Ruiz L, Palascak JB, Gelrud A. Hypertriglyceridemic pancreatitis: presentation and management. *Am J Gastroenterol*. 2009;104(4):984-991.

Valdivielso P, Ramirez-Bueno A, Ewald N. Current knowledge of hypertriglyceridemic pancreatitis. *Eur J Intern Med*. 2014;25(8):689-694.

van der Gaag NA, Rauws EAJ, van Eijck CHJ, et al. Preoperative biliary drainage for cancer of the head of the pancreas. *N Engl J Med*. 2010;362(2):129-137.

van Santvoort HC, Besselink MG, Bakker OJ, et al. A step-up approach or open necrosectomy for necrotizing pancreatitis. *N Engl J Med*. 2010;362(16):1491-1502.

Varadarajulu S, Bang JY, Sutton BS, Trevino JM, Christein JD, Wilcox CM. Equal efficacy of endoscopic and surgical cystogastrostomy for pancreatic pseudocyst drainage in a randomized trial. *Gastroenterology*. 2013;145(3):583-590.

Vinik AI, Woltering EA, Warner RR, et al. NANETS consensus guidelines for the diagnosis of neuroendocrine tumor. *Pancreas*. 2010;39(6):713-734.

Wani AA, Maqsood S, Lala P, Wani S. Annular pancreas in adults: a report of two cases and review of literature. *JOP*. 2013;14(3):277-279.

Williams EJ, Green J, Beckingham I, Parks R, Martin D, Lombard M. Guidelines on the management of common bile duct stones (CBDS). *Gut*. 2008;57(7):1004-1021.

Zheng B, Wang X, Ma B, Tian J, Jiang L, Yang K. Endoscopic stenting versus gastrojejunostomy for palliation of malignant gastric outlet obstruction. *Dig Endosc*. 2012;24(2):71-78.

Zheng ZJ, Gong J, Xiang GM, Mai G, Liu XB. Pancreatic panniculitis associated with acinar cell carcinoma of the pancreas: a case report. *Ann Dermatol*. 2011;23(2):225-228.

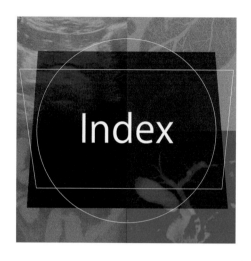

Index

Printed in the United States
by Baker & Taylor Publisher Services